The Perfect Wedding Workout

MICHAEL LIMMER

THE PERFECT wedding WORKOUT

LOOK YOUR BEST
ON THE BIG DAY
IN JUST 10 WEEKS

MEYER & MEYER SPORT

British Library Cataloguing in Publication Data
A catalogue record for this book is available from the British Library

The Perfect Wedding Workout
Maidenhead: Meyer & Meyer Sport (UK) Ltd., 2018
ISBN: 978-1-78255-146-1

© 2018 by Meyer & Meyer Sport (UK) Ltd.
Aachen, Auckland, Beirut, Dubai, Hägendorf, Hong Kong, Indianapolis, Cairo, Cape Town, Manila, Maidenhead, New Delhi, Singapore, Sydney, Teheran, Vienna

🖎 Member of the World Sports Publishers' Association (WSPA)
Printed by Print Consult, GmbH, Munich, Germany

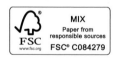

ISBN: 978-1-78255-146-1
Email: info@m-m-sports.com
www.m-m-sports.com

Contents

PHOTO CREDITS

Cover photo:	Photographer Martin Saumweber, Zillertalstudio, Munich
Inside photos:	Avis Wrentmore, Los Angeles
Inside jewelry photos:	© Adobe Stock pages 14, 18, 20, 27, 37, 81, 173, 189, 192, 203, 206, 207, 208, 209, 210, 211, 213
Chapter lead:	© Adobe Stock
Photo of Lara Joy Körner	© Hadley Hudson
Model:	Vanessa Eichholz
Makeup:	Anna Scharl
Costumes bridal gown:	White Silhouette – THE CREATIVE BRIDE, Munich
Cover and interior design:	Annika Naas
Layout:	Ute Kuettner
Managing editors:	Elizabeth Evans and Kristina Oltrogge
Copyeditor:	Anne Rumery

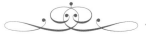

INTRODUCTION

 BY

LARA JOY KÖRNER

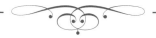

I met Michael on a cold, sunny day in February. The first snowdrops brought with them the promise of spring, and I imagined myself peeling off my thick sweater soon to reveal a slender, strong, energetic body.

I wasn't overweight nor was I entirely unathletic (I had done yoga before), but on a feel-good scale from one to ten with ten being the best, I was a consistent six to seven. I wanted to feel lighter, stronger, and more vigorous, and I wanted to be able to do a freestanding handstand because I had always considered that an expression of freedom and the joy of living. But I also didn't want to get too big; I wanted muscle definition, but not a six-pack.

Michael prescribed eight exercises to be alternated in regular intervals to create a new training stimulus for each workout session. I did these exercises at home every other day. At first, it took me 45 minutes to do the entire workout. After a few weeks, it only took me 22 minutes to do the same number of exercises, so even though the time expenditure was negligible, the training effect was enormous.

By April I already felt great! I had lost weight and could easily carry my heavy grocery bags up the stairs, and multiple women had asked what I did to get such nice upper arms. Isn't that everybody's dream? At the beginning of May—two and a half months later—my feel-good rating was off the charts. The handstand was still a bit shaky, but perfection is overrated.

In a very short amount of time and without great effort, Michael's exercises helped me create an attractive back, nicely defined arms, more endurance, a solid stance, and, because I was so proud of myself, a radiant demeanor.

That is how I want you to feel on your wedding day!

Enjoy creating your personal dream figure.

Lara Joy Körner

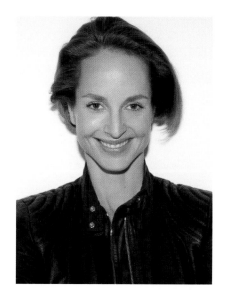

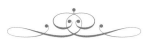

1 PREFACE

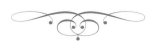

1 Preface

Thank you for choosing *The Perfect Wedding Workout!* I am delighted to accompany you on your path to your perfect wedding figure for the happiest day of your life.

This workout is based on my experience as a personal trainer. The Perfect Wedding Workout is designed to meet the specific requirements for an optimal wedding-day figure to help you achieve the best possible results within a short period of time.

1.1 ABOUT ME

I have been working as a personal trainer on the international level for ten years. I work primarily in Los Angeles, New York, Munich, and Berlin. I frequently train models and actors to get them physically fit for various projects, but I mostly work with women who are weeks away from their wedding and want to feel great on their big day.

I have also worked in the area of therapeutic and health-focused strength training and have experience in performance sports. I have therefore acquainted myself with all areas of professional fitness training and have depth of experience.

1.2 HOW THE PERFECT WEDDING WORKOUT WAS CREATED

My clients are primarily women who are just a few weeks away from their wedding and hire me to work intensively on their wedding figure. Over the course of the past ten years, I have developed a program that will help women achieve their personal dream figure in ten weeks. I have summarized this content for you in *The Perfect Wedding Workout.*

1.3 ADVANTAGES OF THE PERFECT WEDDING WORKOUT

- Varied workouts

- Tried and tested personal-training exercises

- Dietary advice from a physician

- Beauty tips

- 20-35 minutes 3-4x per week

- Less than 3% of your time goes to working out every other day

- Training goal achieved in 10 weeks

- No equipment needed

- Effective, health-oriented, and functional training

- Sculpts and tightens the body

- Boosts metabolism

- Increases well-being

- Increases self-confidence

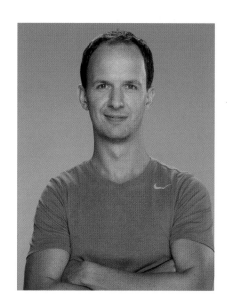

Have fun working out and enjoy a wonderful wedding day with your dream figure!

Michael Limmer

1.4 WHAT IS THE PERFECT WEDDING WORKOUT?

The Perfect Wedding Workout is a workout that brings about three positive changes:

1. Your silhouette

2. Your posture

3. Your gait

It will also improve and have a positive effect on

4. your flexibility

5. your strength, and

6. your endurance.

All of the content is based on my years of experience as a personal trainer. The tried and proven personal-training workouts in this book will guide you to achieve results in just ten weeks, so you can show off your dream figure on the happiest day of your life.

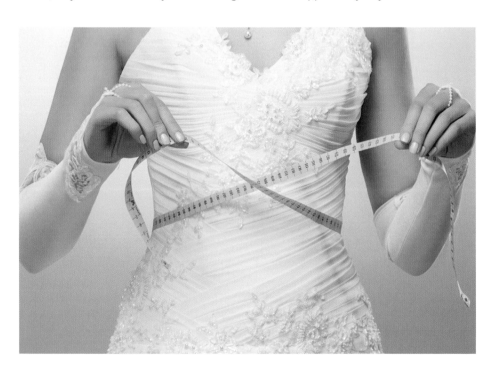

1.5 WHAT MAKES THE PERFECT WEDDING WORKOUT PERFECT?

This program offers effective exercises you need to build your dream figure based on my experience as a personal trainer. Having this book will be like having your own personal trainer in your living room.

Chapter 8 offers nutrition and dietary advice from Dr. Gabriele Anderl, with whom I have had a close working relationship for many years. She will share her substantial knowledge on the complex topic of nutrition, offering clarifications and talking about dietary components that are important to achieving maximum success with the Perfect Wedding Workout.

You will also receive valuable beauty tips from makeup artist Anna Scharl. This book is an all-in-one package that will help you to enjoy the happiest day of your life while looking perfectly beautiful.

1.6 WHAT IS SO SPECIAL ABOUT THE PERFECT WEDDING WORKOUT DIET?

This book does not include a diet. To date, neither Dr. Anderl nor I know of a diet that is effective in the sense that it reduces weight without the so-called yo-yo effect. Chapter 8 talks about an effective dietary principle, which is uncomplicated and can be easily implemented by anyone.

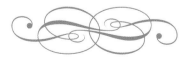

2 MYTHS, MYTHS

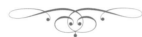 MORE MYTHS

& CLARIFICATION

2 Myths, Myths, More Myths, and Clarification

Nowadays, sports and exercise are major topics. Whether someone goes to a fitness studio, plays a team sport, or is a runner, many who exercise even a little during their free time, tend to think of themselves as experts. Moreover, many glossy magazines and the advertising industry try to influence us with their provocative assertions. Among other things, we are confronted with assertions that are simply not true. Here are ten of the most common myths I have come across, and I am sure they will sound familiar.

#1 More is better.

Wrong! The body needs time to regenerate. For instance, if you work out every day or multiple times a day, you will quickly *overtrain*. You will weaken your immune system, and will actually move farther away from your goals instead of getting closer to them.

#2 You can spot-reduce fat.

Wrong! Some glossy magazines try to make us believe that you just need to do a few sit-ups to lose belly fat and can achieve a six-pack in just three weeks, but it doesn't work that way. Of course abdominal strengthening exercises are important and indispensable, but that does not mean that you are simultaneously reducing belly fat. The body works as a whole;

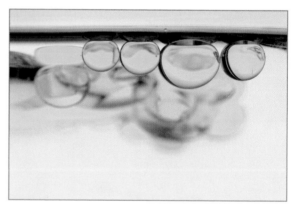

fat can only be reduced on the entire body, and only when we take in fewer calories than we burn (i.e., when we maintain a negative calorie balance).

#3 Fat can be turned into muscle.

Wrong! That doesn't work if for no other reason than the fact that fat and muscle have completely different functions within our bodies. Many who are just starting to exercise lose fat while simultaneously building muscle which doesn't translate to a big difference on the scale. It is important to understand that what matters is what the body is made of and not how heavy it is. Turning fat into muscle is absolutely impossible; apples cannot turn into oranges.

#4 Calories will only begin to burn after 30 minutes.

Wrong! When you exercise, your body works right from the start. Exercise intensity is critical. When you exercise within your comfort zone where you are barely exerting yourself, the exercise will of course be less effective than when you go all out after the warm-up.

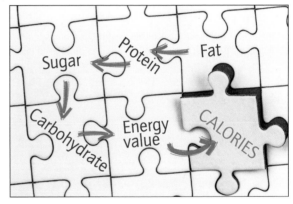

The exercises in the Perfect Wedding Workout will activate your muscle fibers which is the furnace in which you burn the calories. As soon as you increase the amount of active muscle fibers by exercising, they will automatically burn more calories—even as you sleep—and especially during the regeneration phase (i.e., after you finish exercising).

#5 Strength training causes weight gain, and endurance training burns calories.

Wrong! Our muscles work like a furnace in which we burn our calories. When our muscles are active, we automatically burn more calories. First, your skin becomes taut and your belly flattens before you build big muscles. Your calorie balance is responsible for your weight loss. If I want to lose weight, I have to burn more calories than I consume, meaning I have to create a negative calorie balance. On the other hand, if I want to build muscle and gain weight, I need a positive calorie balance.

#6 Building muscle makes you inflexible and inactive.

Wrong! There isn't a sport that doesn't work on muscles and does strictly sport-specific training. And with good reason! As an athlete, you need to be active and flexible. You achieve that with functional interval training.

Another important topic in the Perfect Wedding Workout is stretching. This program will make your muscles supple and sculpt your body.

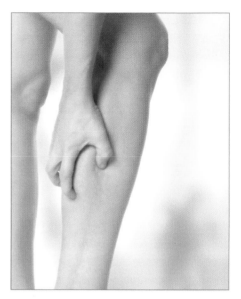

#7 No pain, no gain.

Wrong! Exercise should never cause severe pain. However, your muscles can and should burn, a feeling that many clients refer to as pleasant pain.

#8 If your muscles aren't sore, the exercises aren't effective.

Wrong! Having sore muscles is actually a micro-injury of the muscle fibers. For that reason alone, being sore should never be a training goal. If you do get sore muscles, it's not the end of the world, but it has nothing to do with the effectiveness of an exercise. Muscle soreness usually occurs when you first start to exercise, as well as when the body has to learn new movements and muscular exertions.

#9 Women should only do endurance training.

Wrong! Strength training has a positive effect on your silhouette, gait, posture, and muscles. Endurance training is strength training for the heart and should also be a regular part of your workout. Due to the short breaks, this workout provides the perfect mix of both components.

#10 Eating late causes weight gain.

Wrong! Lots of people who try to lose weight are determined not to eat after 5pm. The theory is that a long break between meals will boost the metabolism, but there is no evidence to back this up. It is the daily and overall intake of calories that determines whether we gain or lose weight. The calories don't care how late it is.

However, if you routinely consume lots of calories late in the evening, it is recommended to eliminate that meal or, if necessary, substitute it with lighter fare.

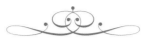

3 EXERCISE PRINCIPLES

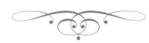

3 Exercise Principles

1. EXERCISE FREQUENCY

Exercise every other day, with a day of regeneration in between.

The training is based on the principle of abbreviated supercompensation.

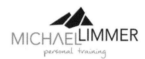

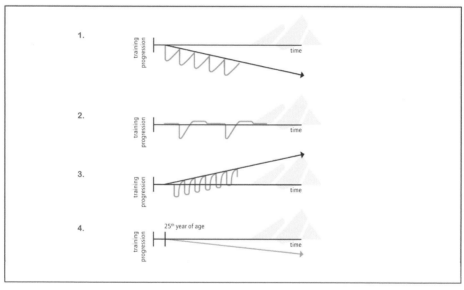

Supercompensation and possible training progressions.

The black line shows the starting level as well as the amount of time.

The green line shows the performance level as well as the training progression.

Generally, we initially weaken the body and the muscles during exercise. After exercising, the body needs time to regenerate to compensate for the exertion, to get stronger, and to get closer to the training goal.

In the above illustration we can see a variety of training progressions:

1) The first shows that a second training impulse was set immediately after the first without observing the important regeneration phase. The result is that you move away from your training goal as you further weaken the body and the muscles. This training progression should never be recommended, but I often see this scenario with overly motivated clients who work out every day or even multiple times a day. I strongly advise against doing so because you may damage your health, and you will not achieve your training goal.

2) The second shows a training progression that is stagnant. The regeneration phases are too long and the next training impulse comes too late. With the Perfect Wedding Workout, you exercise 3-4 times per week with one day of rest between workouts. This day of rest is just as important as the workout itself.

3) The third shows the ideal training progression for your dream figure. You exercise, give your body enough time to regenerate, and then set the next training impulse. It is the only way you will achieve your dream figure. The Perfect Wedding Workout is specifically designed so your body regenerates sufficiently during the 24-hour rest period to be able to vigorously complete the next workout. Recommendations for the ideal way to regenerate can be found on the following pages.

4) The fourth shows the biological degradation process. This means that metabolic activity and active muscle fibers pull back. The result is that we gain weight and our body shape changes in a negative way. In this scenario, the progression of performance capacity looks like the graph under item 4.

2. EXERCISE INTENSITY

The first two weeks are used to acclimate at submaximal intensity. After that, let your muscles burn and work out until you reach *localized muscle exhaustion*. To build your dream body, you need an above-threshold stimulus. That means: You do as many repetitions or hold a position as long as you can. As you do so, think about the goal you set: to make your wedding gown shine with your dream figure. It is not the length of the workout but the intensity that determines the success of the workout.

3. THE AFTERBURN EFFECT

Utilize the afterburn effect! It is now an undisputed fact that intensive interval training burns the most calories. After a workout, the core temperature and the pulse are elevated and the energy stores must be refilled. That means that, even after a workout, the body still works hard to return to its normal state. A US study* proves that the afterburn effect can last for up to 14 hours after a workout, meaning that you are still actively burning additional calories during that period of time. To make the most of the afterburn effect, consume some protein as soon as possible, hydrate, and take a contrast shower (i.e., shower in warm/hot water for 3-5 minutes, and then immediately after, turn on the cold water for 1 minute only). Then lie down for 10-15 minutes with your legs elevated and rest.

4. BREAKS

Take short breaks between exercises. Look for recommendations under "Performance Level" in the next chapter. Get a drink of water and go right back to your workout. Long breaks make your workout ineffective. You can take a well-deserved break after the workout.

5. BREATHING

During intensive training units, it is important that the body gets enough oxygen. That means avoiding exhaling on exertion and not holding your breath. Try to breathe evenly.

6. HYDRATION

Drink sufficient amounts of water before, during, and after you work out. Avoid sugar and minimize alcohol consumption. Independent of working out, you should never wait until you are thirsty to hydrate. Water is our fuel. Just like a car cannot drive without fuel, our body cannot work productively without water.

> *Your formula for fluid consumption is approximately 35 ml per kg of bodyweight. If you weigh 70 kg, you should consume 2.45 liters of fluid, preferably water.*

*Study done at the University of Colorado-Denver and published in "Exercise and Sport Science Review," 2009.

7. QUALITY OF EXECUTION

Good form should never be compromised. As soon as you notice that you are no longer able to execute the exercise as prescribed, discontinue the exercise and instead try to do the same exercise longer during the next workout. Performing an exercise incorrectly is not conducive to reaching the training goal.

8. CONTRAST SHOWERS

Take a contrast shower after every workout. It is an active regeneration method. It speeds up regeneration while also boosting metabolism and circulation. After showering with warm water for approximately 30 seconds, gradually reduce the water temperature until the water is so cold that you can just tolerate it. Keep the water at this temperature for 20-30 seconds, then turn the water temperature back to warm. Repeat this process for 5-8 minutes. By the way, contrast showers are said to also be effective against cellulite, and many of my clients confirm this.

9. MOTIVATION

Stay motivated and don't give in to your inner couch potato. You are stronger! Stay focused on your goal! For instance, take a photo of your dream dress and use it as a screen saver on your laptop and smartphone. Write your ideal measurements on a mirror with lipstick to keep your eye on the prize. Tell your friends and coworkers about your plan. It is important to always remember your goal.

If you stick to these basic principles and complete the Perfect Wedding Workout, nothing will keep you from reaching your personal goal and fully enjoying the happiest day of your life wearing your dream figure.

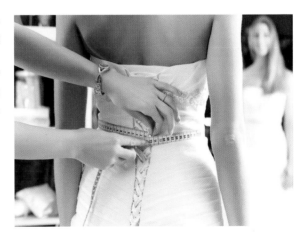

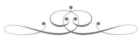

4 INSTRUCTION MANUAL

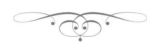

4 Instruction Manual

4.1 FREQUENTLY ASKED QUESTIONS

- Interval training? Circuit training? What is that?

  The Perfect Wedding Workout is an interval training program with effective exercises to achieve your ideal bridal figure. The workout is completed in a circuit. It helps you sculpt your body, activate the muscles, and, due to the short breaks, it also boosts the metabolism. During the highly intensive workout phase, your body requires more oxygen, and metabolic function increases greatly. More energy is needed to return the body to its normal state during the subsequent break. The constant ramping up and down of your "engine" results in the body's continued burning of calories long after the actual workout. The keyword is the afterburn effect.

- How can I be more active in my daily life?

  Try to take 8,500-10,000 steps per day. You can use a pedometer to keep track. Most of us only take 2,000-4,500 steps per day. Think of your goal. In addition to the workout, an active lifestyle is very important. You can achieve this high number of steps by:

  - Not sitting or lying down while **talking on the phone**. Walk around your apartment or house. Go up and down steps. If you use a smartphone, walk around outside.

  - **Parking your car** far away from the entrance to the grocery store and not right in front of the door.

  - **Using public transportation** on your way to work. Get off one or two stops sooner and walk the rest of the way.

  - **Using the stairs** instead of the elevator or escalator.

  - By going to see your **colleague next door** rather than calling him when you have a question.

  - By taking a quick walk during your lunch break.

- How long should the breaks be between exercises?

Each person has an individual performance capacity and an individual performance level. The book offers recommendations for breaks based on my experience as a personal trainer. However, you can modify the breaks on your own.

Important: A break should never be longer than 30 seconds!!!

 Use a timer to train effectively!

Performance level 1

Has never exercised, hasn't exercised in a long time, or does less than 1 hour of exercise per week.

Recommended break length: 20 seconds

Performance level 2

Casual exerciser, 1-3 hours per week max.

Recommended break length: 20 seconds

Performance level 3

Exercises regularly, 3 hours or more per week.

Recommended break length: 15 seconds

- **How hard do I have to exercise?**

  You need to experience localized muscle exhaustion during your final set. That means you need to do each exercise until you are unable to do another repetition with the correct form. The muscles need to burn. That is the only way you will achieve the above-threshold stimulus that will take you one step closer to your dream figure. Every performance level has a certain time allowance for each exercise. I have determined these time allowances as guidelines based on my experience. Though they apply perfectly to the vast majority of exercisers, each person is unique. If you notice that the time allowance doesn't meet your capacity, you can and should exceed it.

Important: The exercises should never hurt!

 Stay completely focused on your workout and don't allow anything to distract you during that period of time. Also, actively tighten the muscles you are working to achieve the maximum effect!!

- **How can I stay motivated?**

  In order to stay truly motivated for the ten weeks, all of my future brides—without exception—sign the contract below. You need to place this workout contract in a highly visible place, ideally some place where you will see it several times a day (e.g., your bathroom mirror, in the car, at work, or even as a background photo on your smartphone, tablet, or laptop).

- **Which exercises do I need to complete?**

  In chapter 6 you will find out which exercises you will need to complete. The workouts are versatile, and the structure and exercise sequence are pre-planned for each training week. They are highly effective and based on my many years of personal-training experience. Many of my clients achieved their dream figure by adhering to these plans.

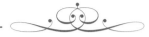

Workout Contract
THE PERFECT WEDDING WORKOUT

Name: _____

Trainer: Michael Limmer

Training period: 10 weeks

Start date: _____

Wedding date: _____

Workout location: At home, in the backyard, or at the park

Training goal: My ideal bridal figure on my wedding day

_____

_____

_____

_____

I hereby pledge to implement the content of *The Perfect Wedding Workout* by Michael Limmer and to consistently exercise to achieve my ideal bridal figure.

Date, Place _____

Signature of Exerciser _____

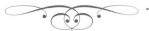

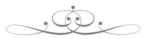

5 REGENERATION

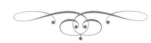

5 Regeneration

Regeneration is an important part of the Perfect Wedding Workout. Before we move on to the exercises and the workout, I would like to introduce a few effective regeneration methods. Along with exercise and nutrition, *regeneration* is another important factor to ensure effective exercise. You can significantly lower the risk of muscle soreness if you regenerate consciously and consistently.

1. **Sleep!** As trite as it may sound, sleep is the basis for regeneration. Only while you sleep do your brain and your muscles relax completely. This rest is important; it allows you to be productive again afterwards. Sleep requirements vary. Seven hours has proven effective for many of my clients. A 20-30 minute nap during the day, if possible, is also recommended.

2. **Massages.** Let your partner give you a massage. Massages are therapeutic and relax the body and mind. And your partner will most likely enjoy it, too! Of course you can also make an appointment with a physical therapist or massage therapist.

3. **Stretching.** Stretching can relieve tension and makes muscles supple. In the following chapter, you will find out which stretches are useful.

4. **Contrast showers.** As previously mentioned, contrast showers are an integral part of the Perfect Wedding Workout.

5. **Diet.** And not just any diet, but the right one. You will find out what that looks like when you read the nutrition chapter by Dr. Gabriele Anderl.

6. **Water.** Pay attention to your water intake. We recommend 35 ml per kg of body weight. Try to have a bottle of water within reach at all times. Put a bottle in your car, have a bottle ready at your workplace, and ideally start your fluid intake at breakfast.

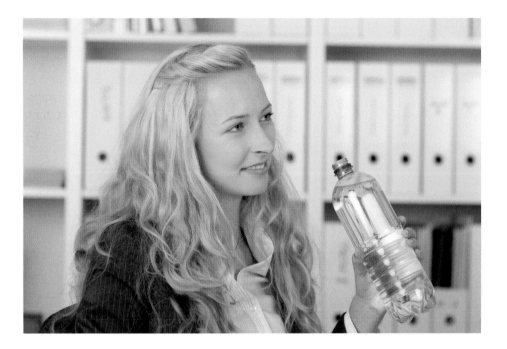

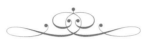

6 EXERCISES

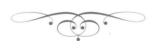

6 Exercises

6.1 UPPER BODY AND CORE

Shadowboxing

Stand in a stable straddle stance and punch across your body, alternating arms (i.e., move the left arm to the right and the right arm to the left). Gradually increase the tempo and adhere to the specified amount of time. Try to achieve maximum speed before the time is up.

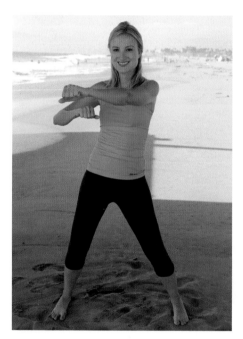
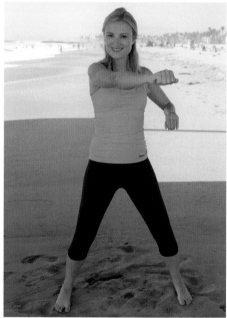

Standing crunch

Bring one knee and the opposite elbow together at the center of the body. Try to keep your movements fluid.

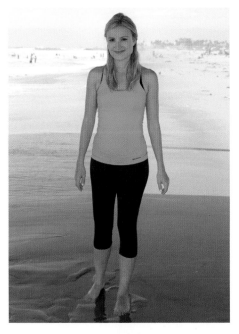

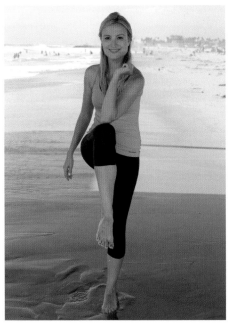

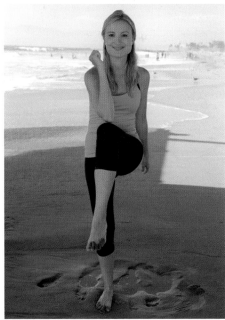

45-degree push-ups

Get into push-up position against a wall. Hands are shoulder-width apart against the wall, legs are extended, and the back is straight. Keeping your body straight, try to get as close to the wall as you can. Make sure to maintain body tension.

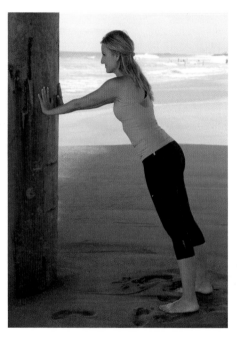 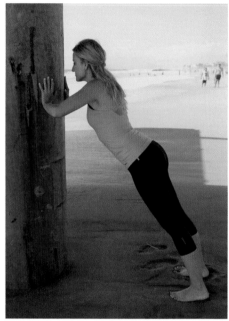

45-degree three-point push-ups

Get into push-up position against a wall. Hands are shoulder-width apart against the wall, legs are extended, and the back is straight. Now lift one leg off the ground and try to get as close to the wall as possible while keeping the body straight. Make sure to maintain body tension.

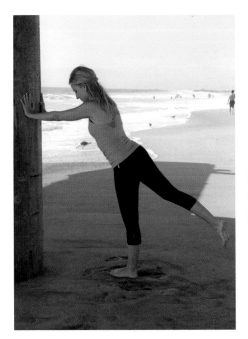 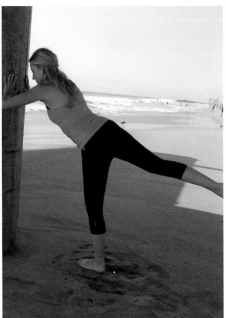

Kneeling push-ups

Get into a kneeling push-up position. Cross your ankles and keep your upper body stable; hands are shoulder-width apart. Now lower the upper body as far as possible while keeping your back straight. Make sure your back is straight and the head is an extension of the spine.

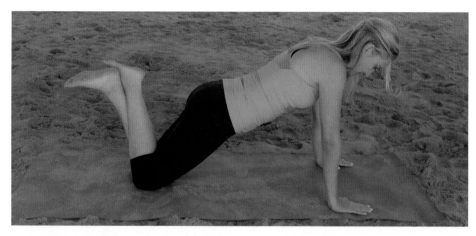

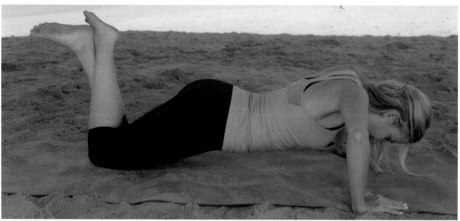

Kneeling three-point push-ups

Get into a kneeling push-up position and extend one leg horizontally behind you. Hands are shoulder-width apart. Now alternate raising the extended leg while lowering the upper body as much as you can with a straight back. Make sure the back is straight and the head is an extension of the spine.

Important: Actively tighten your stomach and trunk muscles.

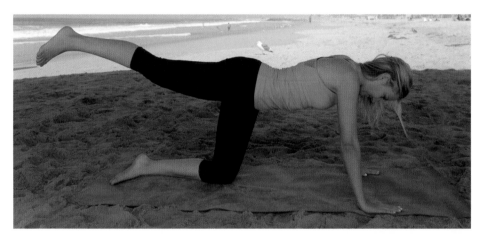

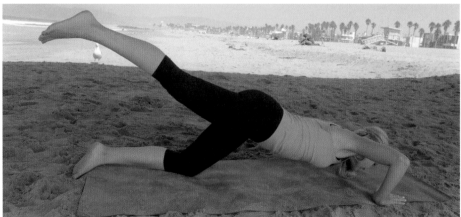

Classic push-ups

Get into a classic push-up position with hands shoulder-width apart. Now get as low as possible while keeping your upper body straight. Make sure the back is straight and the head is an extension of the spine.

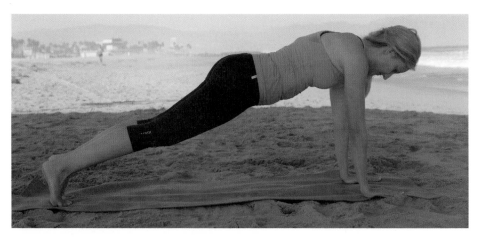

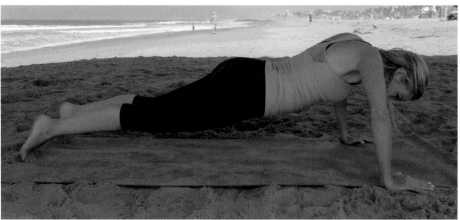

Push-up position + forward extension

The starting position is the push-up position. Hold an additional weight (e.g., bottle of water, book, purse) in one hand. Now extend that arm as far forward as you can without changing the position of your core (center of the body). To do so, actively tighten the core muscles and focus on the arm movement.

Important: Work both sides!

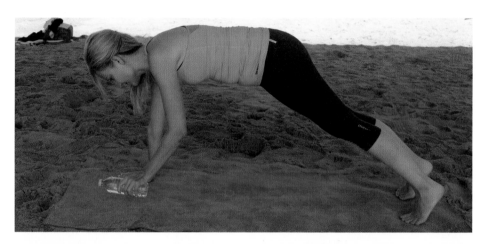

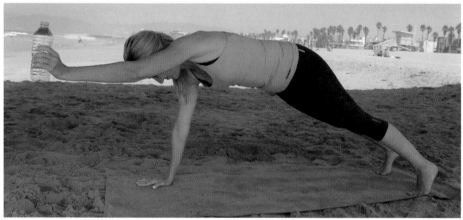

90-degree dips

Sit in a chair and grip the chair close to the body with your elbows pointing backward, opposite the direction of your gaze. Legs are bent 90 degrees. Now scoot forward a little so only your arms and legs bear your bodyweight. Next lower your bottom as far as you can while bending your elbows. Immediately after, shift your center of gravity up again and straighten the arms.

Important: The back remains straight, the head is always an extension of the spine, and the elbows always point backward.

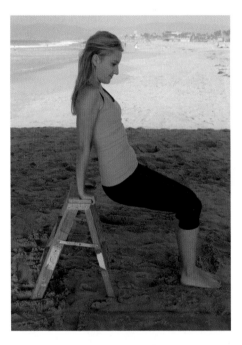 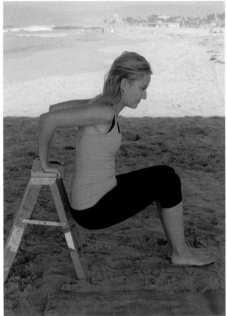

Push-up position + lateral extension

The starting position is the push-up position. Hold an additional weight (e.g., bottle of water, book, purse) in one hand. Now extend that arm to the side and up without changing the position of your core (center of the body). To do so, tighten the muscles of the trunk and focus on the arm movement.

Important: Work both sides!

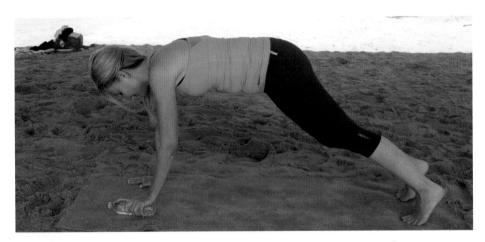

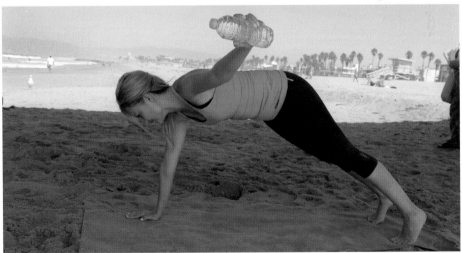

Parachutist push-ups

First get into classic push-up position. Now raise the hips as high as you can and move your toes about a foot's length closer to your hands. In this position, bend your elbows and lower your head toward the ground, and if possible barely touch the ground with your forehead. Next, straighten the arms and return to the starting position.

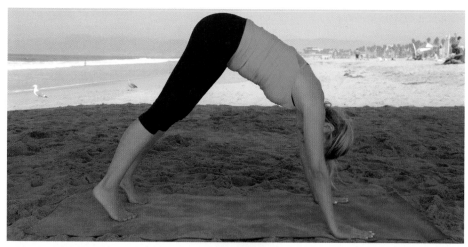

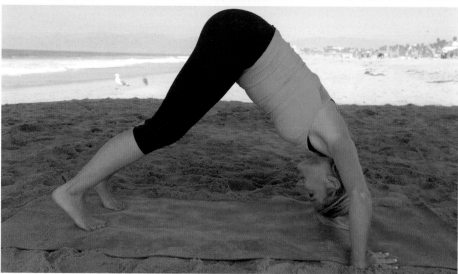

Extended dips

Sit in a chair and grip the chair close to the body with your elbows pointing backward, opposite the direction of your gaze. Legs are extended. Scoot forward a little so your arms and feet support all of your weight. Now bend your elbows and try to lower your bottom as much as possible. Immediately after, shift your center of gravity up again and straighten the arms.

Important: The back remains straight, the head is always an extension of the spine, and the elbows point backward.

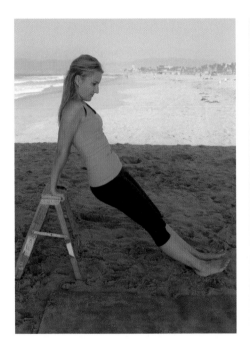
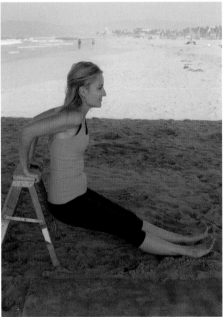

Three-point dips

Sit in a chair and grip the chair close to the body with your elbows pointing backward, opposite the direction of your gaze. Legs are extended. Scoot forward a little so your arms support all of your weight, and lift one leg. Now bend your elbows and try to lower your bottom as much as possible. Immediately after, shift your center of gravity up again and straighten the arms.

Important: *The back remains straight, the head is always an extension of the spine, and the elbows point backward.*

Important: *Work both sides!*

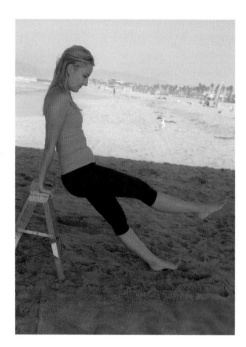
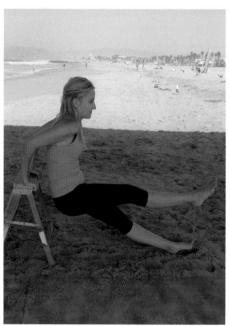

Arm extension on your side

Lie on your side with your shoulder resting on the ground and your legs and hips stacked. Lay your lower arm across your ribcage and place the hand of the upper arm on the ground in front of the sternum. Now use your upper arm to raise your upper body off the ground as much as you can.

Important: *Work both sides!*

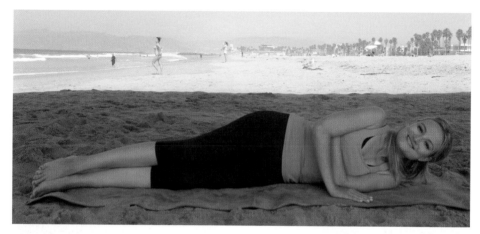

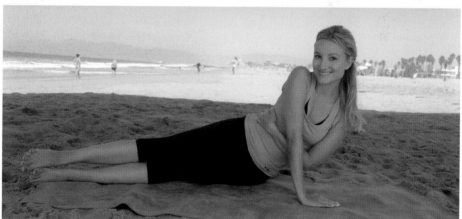

Kneeling forearm plank + leg extension

During this exercise the body is supported by the knees and forearms. Keep your mid-section steady. Actively tighten your abdominal muscles and avoid arching or rounding your back. The head is an extension of the spine. Now extend one leg straight back in a horizontal position. The leg is an extension of the body. Don't let the body tilt left or right.

Important: Work both sides!

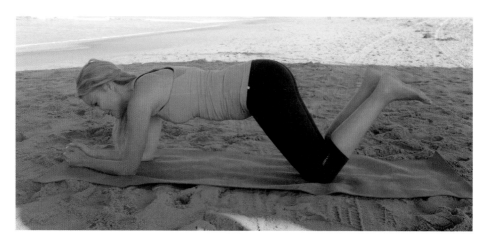

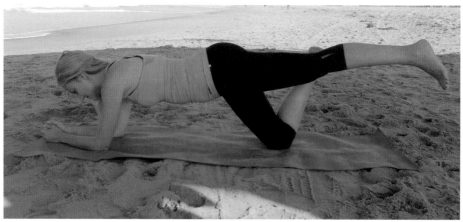

Kneeling forearm plank + diagonal extension

During this exercise the body is supported by the knees and forearms. Keep your midsection steady. Actively tighten your abdominal muscles and avoid arching or rounding your back. The head is an extension of the spine. Now extend one arm forward in a horizontal position and extend the opposite leg back in a horizontal position. The arm is held at head-level, and the leg is an extension of the body. Don't let the body tilt left or right.

Important: Work both sides!

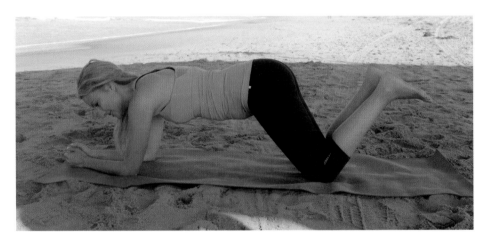

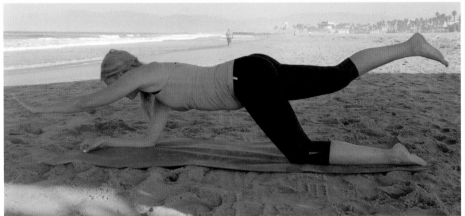

Kneeling forearm plank + arm extension

During this exercise, the body is supported by the knees and forearms. Cross your ankles and keep your midsection steady. Actively tighten your abdominal muscles and avoid arching or rounding your back. The head is an extension of the spine. Now extend one arm forward in a horizontal position. The arm is held at head-level. Don't let the body tilt left or right.

Important: *Work both sides!*

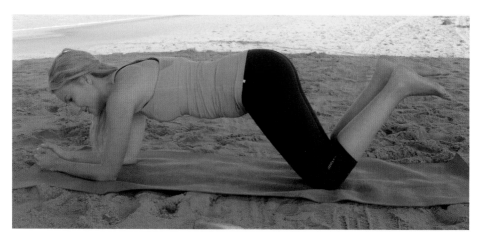

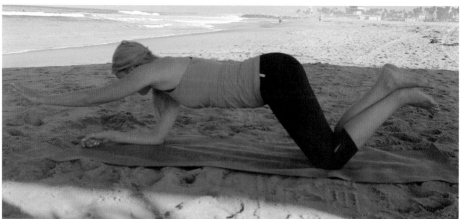

Forearm plank

Your entire body is supported by your forearms. Your back is straight. Do not arch or round your back. The head is an extension of the spine. Try to actively tighten your abdominal muscles.

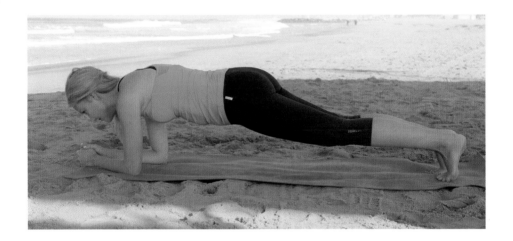

Forearm plank + leg extension

Get into forearm plank position. Remember that your body forms a straight line, the trunk is steady, and your back is neither arched nor rounded. The head is an extension of the spine. Actively tighten your abdominal muscles and maintain that tension. Now lift one leg, keeping the leg extended. Make sure your middle doesn't tilt left or right. Keep the body in a straight line.

Important: Work both sides!

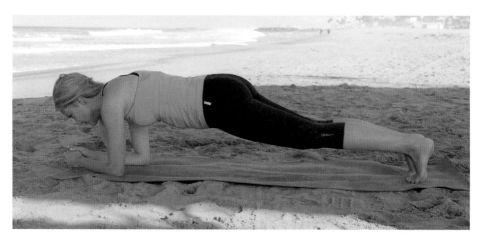

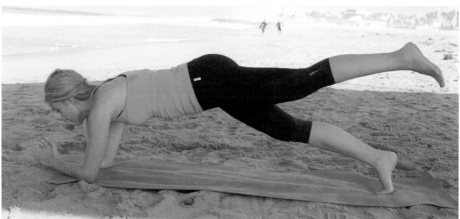

Forearm plank + arm extension

Keep your body in a straight line while alternately lifting one arm into a horizontal position without turning the body to the left or right. The arm is straight and held at head-level. The head is an extension of the spine. Maintain tension in the abdominal muscles.

Important: Work both sides!

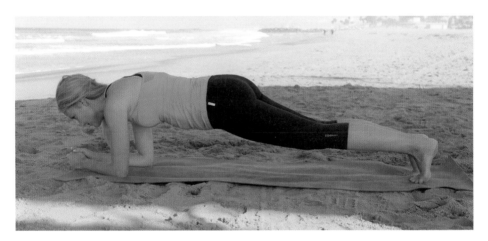

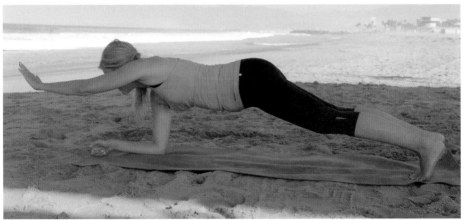

Forearm plank + diagonal extension

Keep your body in a straight line while extending one leg and the opposite arm into a horizontal position without turning the body to the left or right. Your leg and the opposite arm are fully extended and are an extension of the spine, as is the head. Maintain tension in the abdominal muscles.

Important: Work both sides!

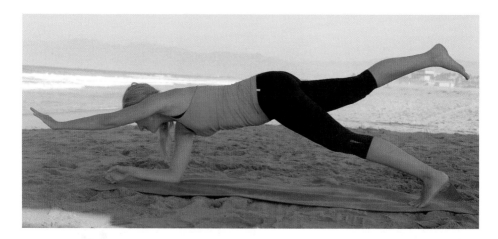

Full plank

Get into push-up position. Make sure your body forms a straight line, the trunk is steady, and the back is neither arched nor rounded. The head is an extension of the spine. Actively tighten your abdominal muscles and maintain that tension.

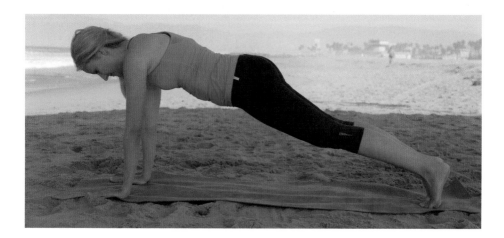

Full plank + leg extension

Get into push-up position. Make sure your body forms a straight line, the trunk is steady, and the back is neither arched nor rounded. The head is an extension of the spine. Actively tighten your abdominal muscles and maintain that tension. Now raise one extended leg. Make sure that your middle doesn't tilt to the left or right. Keep the body in a straight line.

Important: Work both sides!

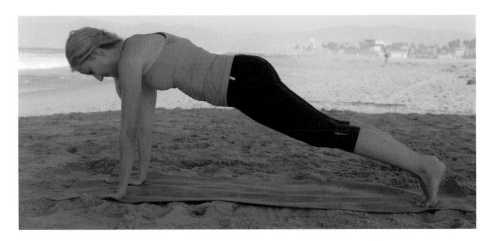

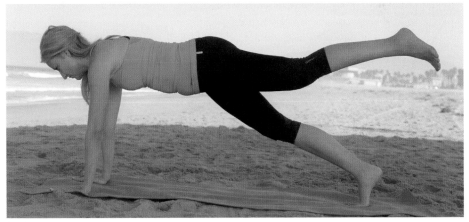

Full plank + arm extension

Get into push-up position. Make sure your body forms a straight line, the trunk is steady, and the back is neither arched nor rounded. Actively tighten your abdominal muscles and maintain that tension. Now raise one arm. Make sure that your middle doesn't tilt to the left or right. Keep the body in a straight line.

Important: *Work both sides!*

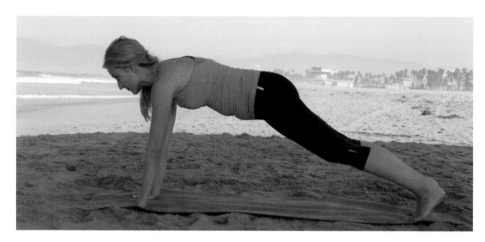

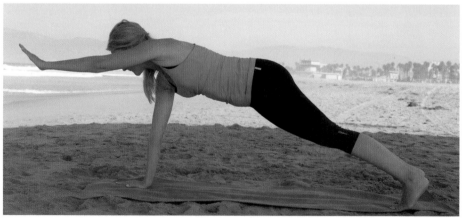

Full plank + diagonal extension

Get into push-up position. Make sure your body forms a straight line, the trunk is steady, and the back is neither arched nor rounded. The head is an extension of the spine. Actively tighten your abdominal muscles and maintain that tension. Now extend one leg behind you and raise the opposite arm. Make sure that your middle doesn't tilt to the left or right. Keep the body in a straight line.

Important: Work both sides!

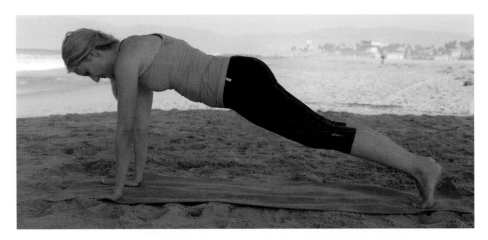

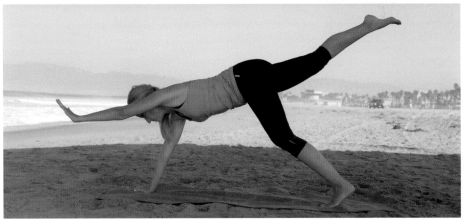

Kneeling forearm side plank

Start by getting on your side. In this exercise, the body rests on your knee and forearm. The knees are bent. Now raise your hips as high as you can while extending the upper arm overhead as far as you can to straighten your hip as much as possible. The body doesn't tilt forward or back, and the head is an extension of the spine. Actively tighten your abdominal muscles.

Important: Work both sides!

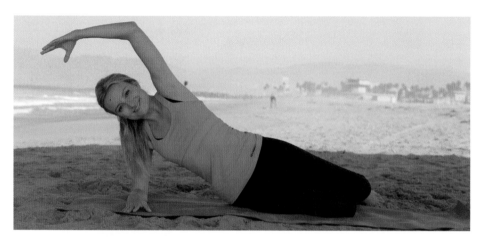

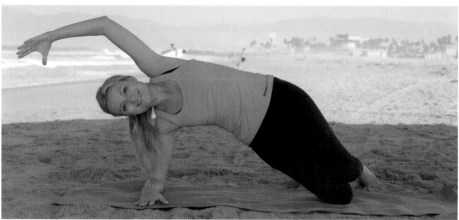

Kneeling forearm side plank + leg extension

Start by getting on your side. In this exercise, the body rests on your knee and forearm. The knees are bent. Now raise your hips as high as you can while extending the upper arm overhead as far as you can to straighten your hip as much as possible. The body doesn't tilt forward or back, and the head is an extension of the spine. Actively tighten your abdominal muscles. Now also lift the upper leg as high as you can. As you do so, make sure to maintain maximum hip extension.

Important: Work both sides!

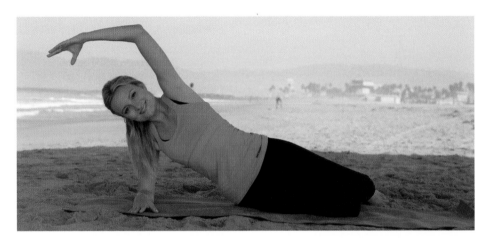

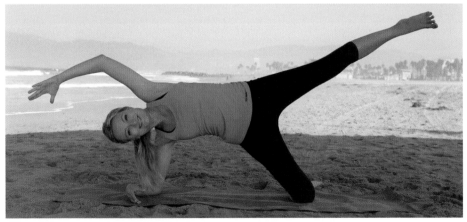

Kneeling forearm side plank + crunch

Start by getting on your side. In this exercise, the body rests on your knee and forearm. The knees are bent. Now raise your hips as high as you can while extending the upper arm overhead as far as you can to straighten your hip as much as possible. The body doesn't tilt forward or back, and the head is an extension of the spine. Actively tighten your abdominal muscles. Now also lift the upper leg as high as you can. As you do so, make sure to maintain maximum hip extension. Now do a crunch by bringing the upper elbow and the upper knee together at the center of the body before returning to the starting position.

Important: Work both sides!

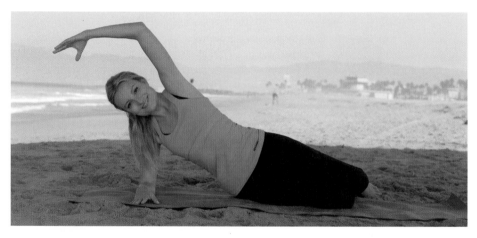

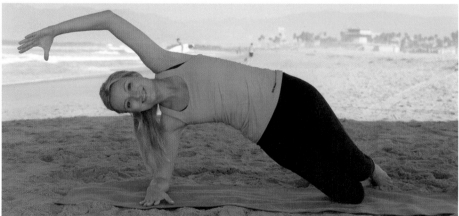

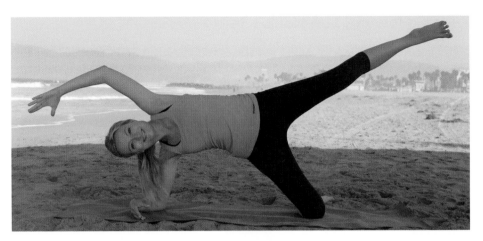

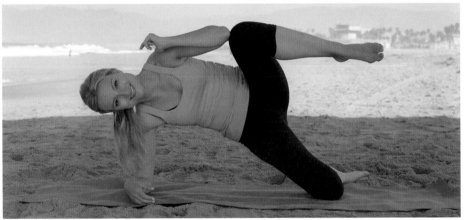

Kneeling forearm side plank + twist

Start by getting on your side. In this exercise, the body rests on your knee and forearm. The knees are bent. Now raise your hips as high as you can while extending the upper arm overhead as far as you can to straighten your hip as much as possible. The body doesn't tilt forward or back, and the head is an extension of the spine. Actively tighten your abdominal muscles. As soon as you are in a stable position, perform a twist by moving the extended arm toward the lower elbow. To do so, you have to internally rotate your body. Try to bring your elbows as close together as possible.

Important: Work both sides!

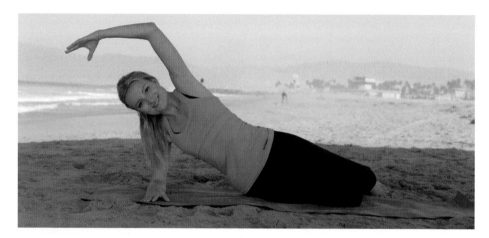

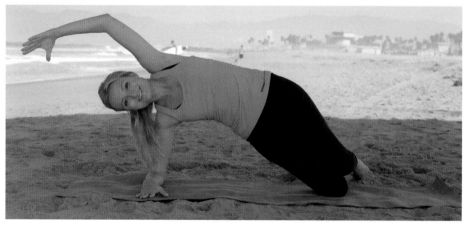

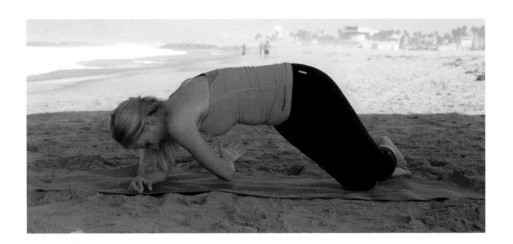

Extended forearm side plank

Start by getting on your side. In this exercise, the body rests on your foot and forearm. Now raise your hips as high as you can while extending the upper arm overhead as far as you can to straighten your hip as much as possible. The body doesn't tilt forward or back, and the head is an extension of the spine. Actively tighten your abdominal muscles.

Important: Work both sides!

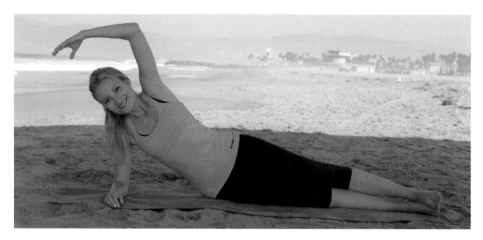

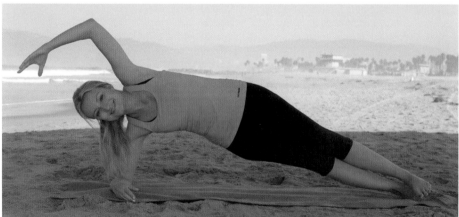

Extended forearm side plank + leg raise

Start by getting on your side. In this exercise, the body rests on your foot and forearm. Now raise your hips as high as you can while extending the upper arm overhead as far as you can to straighten your hip as much as possible. Now raise the top leg as high as possible. The body doesn't tilt forward or back, and the head is an extension of the spine. Actively tighten your abdominal muscles.

Important: *Work both sides!*

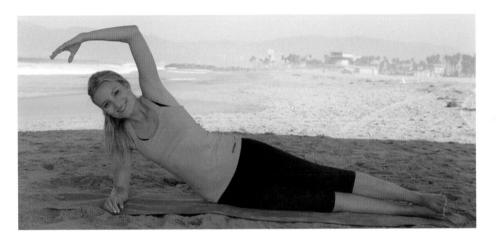

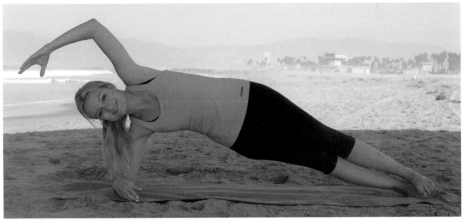

(continued)

Extended forearm side plank + leg raise (continued)

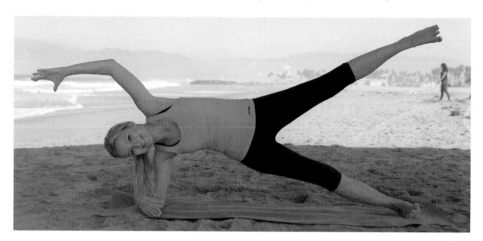

Extended forearm side plank + twist

Start by getting on your side. In this exercise, the body rests on your foot and forearm. Now raise your hips as high as you can while extending the upper arm overhead as far as you can to straighten your hip as much as possible. The body doesn't tilt forward or back, and the head is an extension of the spine. Actively tighten your abdominal muscles. As soon as you are in a stable position, perform a twist by moving the extended arm toward the lower elbow. To do so, you have to internally rotate your body. Try to bring your elbows as close together as possible.

Important: *Work both sides!*

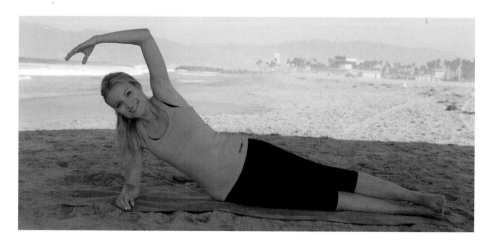

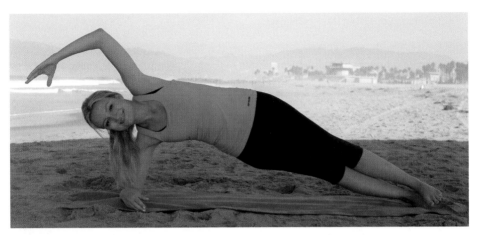

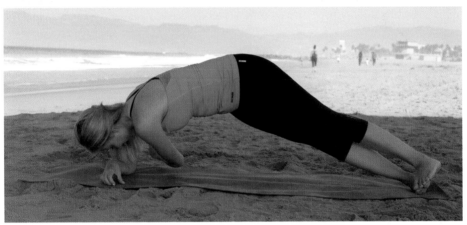

Forearm side-plank + crunch

Start by getting on your side. In this exercise, the body rests on your foot and forearm. Now raise your hips as high as you can while extending the upper arm overhead as far as you can to straighten your hip as much as possible. The body doesn't tilt forward or back, and the head is an extension of the spine. Actively tighten your abdominal muscles. Now also lift the upper leg as high as you can. As you do so, make sure to maintain maximum hip extension. Now do a crunch by bringing the upper elbow and the upper knee together at the center of the body before returning to the starting position.

Important: Work both sides!

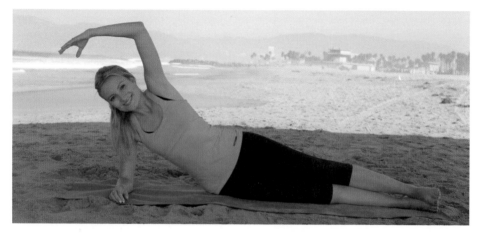

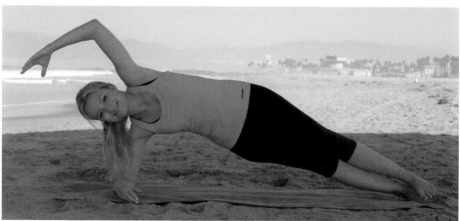

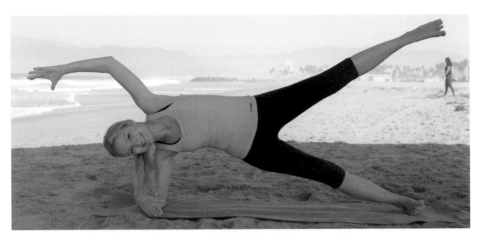

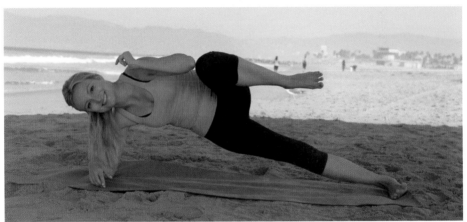

Kneeling shoulder tap

The starting position is a kneeling push-up position. Keep your body straight and maintain body tension by actively tightening your muscles. Now lift one hand off the ground and tap the opposite shoulder. Do a slow repetition.

Important: *Switch sides and keep your middle perfectly straight without shifting your weight to the left or right.*

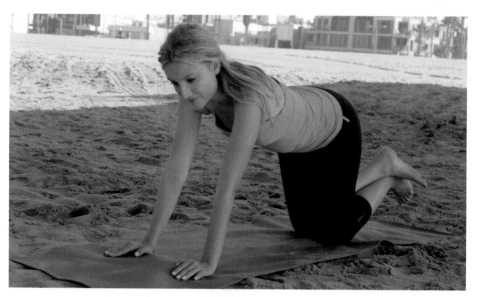

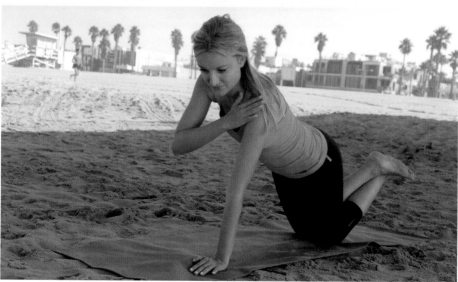

Shoulder tap

The starting position is a push-up position. Keep your body straight and maintain body tension by actively tightening your muscles. Now lift one hand off the ground and tap the opposite shoulder. Do a slow repetition.

Important: Switch sides and keep your middle perfectly straight without shifting your weight to the left or right.

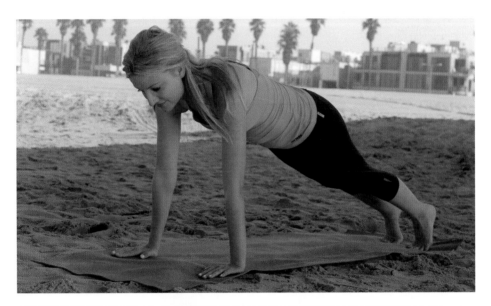

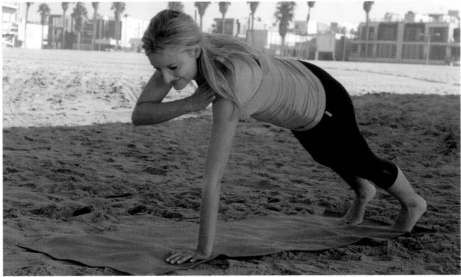

Mountain climber

The starting position is a push-up position. Keep your shoulders as steady as possible and actively tighten your muscles. Now alternate moving each knee as far forward between your arms as possible. As you do so, actively engage your abdominal muscles. The farther forward you can move the knee, the better. Lift the knee and the foot as far off the ground as possible.

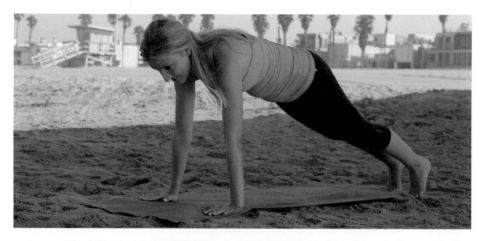

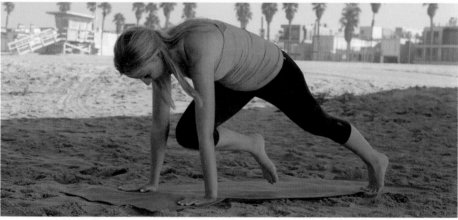

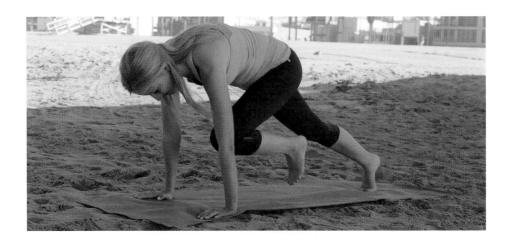

Diagonal mountain climber

The starting position is a push-up position. Keep your shoulders as steady as possible and actively tighten your muscles. Now alternate moving each knee diagonally forward between your arms as far as you can. If possible, touch the knee to the opposite elbow. As you complete the exercise, actively engage your abdominal muscles. The farther forward you can move the knee, the better. Lift the knee and the foot as far off the ground as possible.

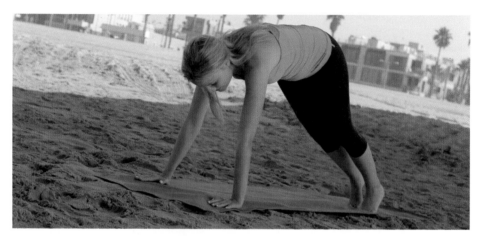

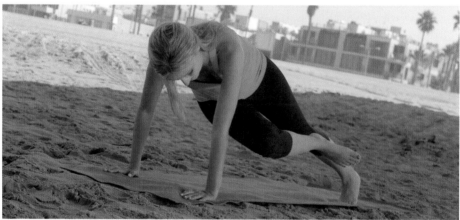

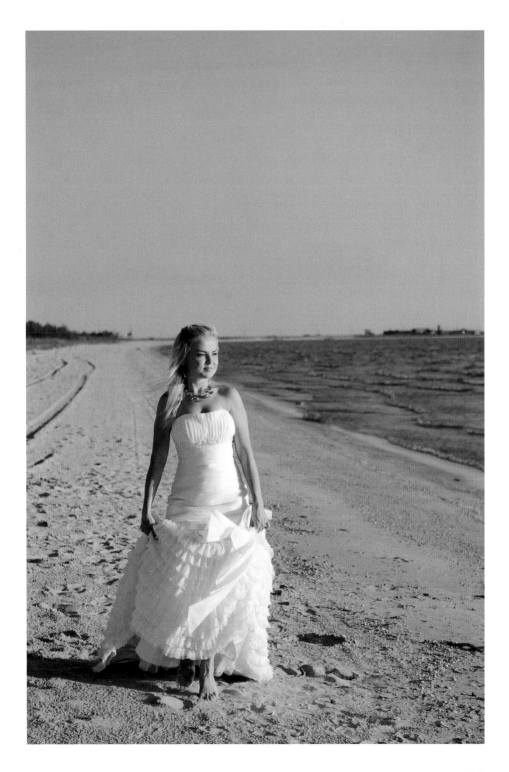

Diagonal bridge crunch

Get into bridge position. Now lift your hips high. The head is initially an extension of the spine. Now move into a crunch and bring one foot and the opposite hand together. Then return to the starting position. Movements should be slow and controlled.

Important: Work both sides!

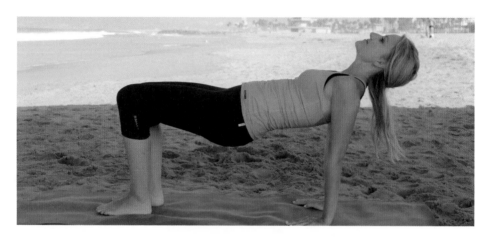

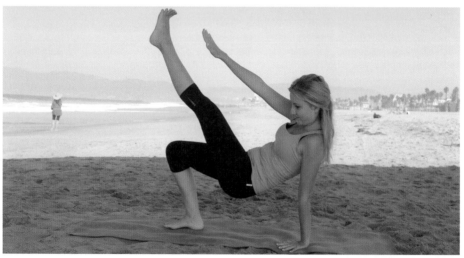

Bridge crunch

Get into bridge position. Now lift your hips high. The head is initially an extension of the spine. Now move into a crunch and bring one foot and the same-side hand together. Then return to the starting position. Movements should be slow and controlled.

Important: *Work both sides!*

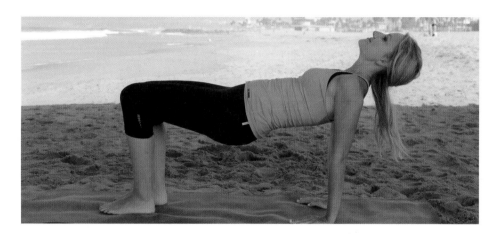

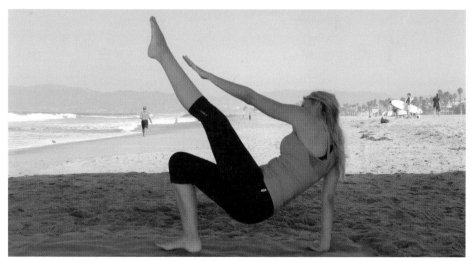

Seated crunch

In a seated position, lean back slightly. Knees are bent and heels are on the ground. Now lean back as far as you can. As you do so, make sure your abdominals are actively engaged. The head is always an extension of the spine.

Now move only your upper body side to side while moving your fingertips as far to the side and away from the body as possible and make brief contact with the ground.

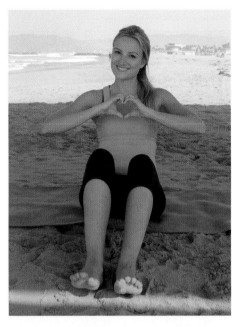

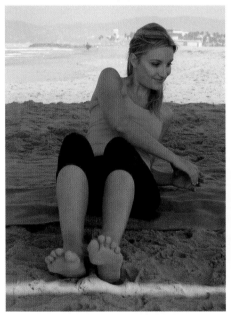

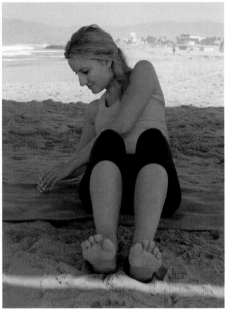

Advanced seated crunch

In a seated position, lean back slightly. Knees are bent and heels are raised at least 5 cm off the ground. Now lean back as far as you can. As you do so, make sure your abdominal muscles are actively engaged. The head is always an extension of the spine.

Now move only your upper body side to side while moving your fingertips as far to the side and away from the body as possible and make brief contact with the ground.

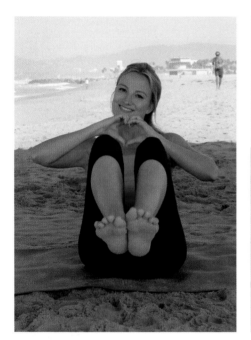 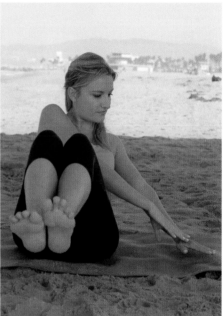

All-fours position + arm extension

Get on all fours. Make sure your back is straight, actively engage your abdominal muscles, and keep your head as an extension of the spine. Now alternately extend the arms forward into a horizontal position without letting the body tilt left or right. The arm is held at head-level. Maintain tension of the abdominal muscles.

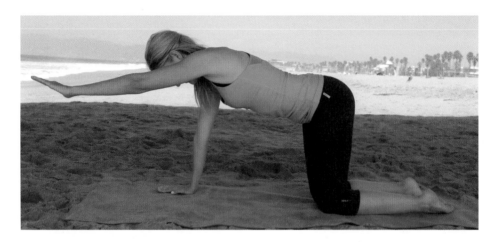

All-fours position + leg extension

Get on all fours. Make sure your back is straight, actively engage your abdominal muscles, and keep your head as an extension of the spine. Now alternately extend the legs backward into a horizontal position without letting the body tilt left or right. The extended leg is an extension of the body axis. Maintain tension of the abdominal muscles.

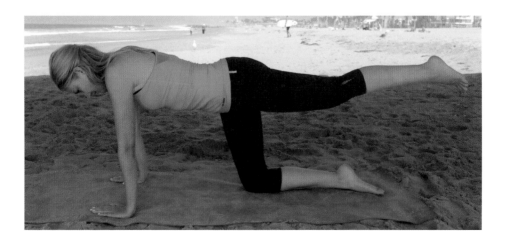

All-fours position + diagonal extension

Get on all fours. Make sure your back is straight, actively engage your abdominal muscles, and keep your head as an extension of the spine. Now alternately extend one leg backward into a horizontal position while extending the opposite arm forward without letting the body tilt left or right. The extended leg is an extension of the body axis; the extended arm is at head-level. Maintain tension of the abdominal muscles.

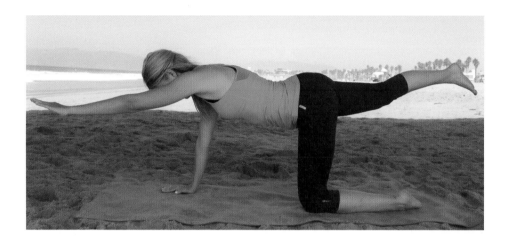

Diagonal all-fours position + crunch

Get on all fours. Make sure your back is straight, actively engage your abdominal muscles, and keep your head as an extension of the spine. Now alternately extend one leg backward into a horizontal position while extending the opposite arm forward without letting the body tilt left or right. The extended leg is an extension of the body axis; the extended arm is at head-level. Now complete a crunch by bringing knee and elbow together in the middle. Maintain tension of the abdominal muscles.

Important: Work both sides!

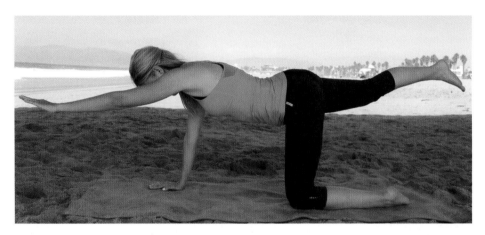

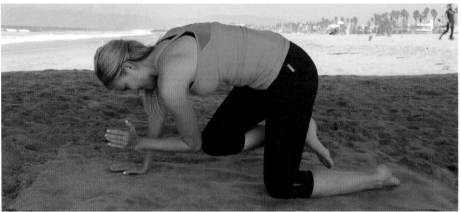

Triceps stretch

Extend one arm up as an extension of your body. Place your free hand on the elbow and try to push the extended arm as far as possible behind your head to feel a stretch in the triceps.

Important: Stretch both sides!

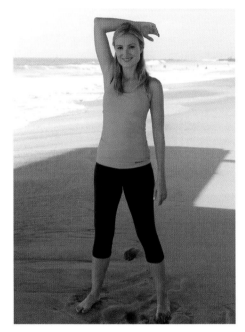
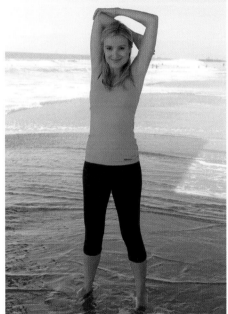

Shoulder stretch

Place one hand across the opposite shoulder. The elbow is parallel to the ground. With your free hand, push the arm as far back as possible.

Important: Stretch both sides!

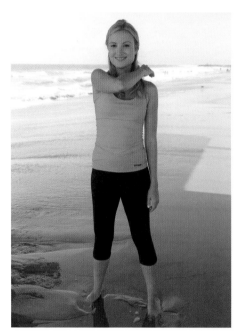
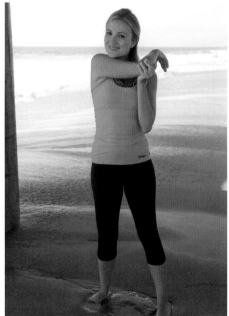

Gluteal stretch

Stand tall. Lift one knee, grip it with both hands, and pull it as close to the chest as possible. Try to achieve a final position in which you can feel a stretch in your gluteal muscles.

Important: Stretch both sides!

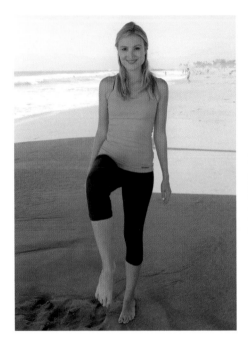 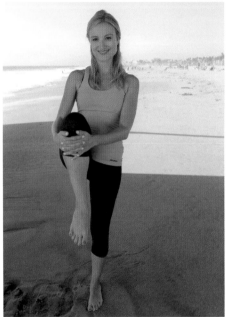

Child's pose

Get on your knees, sit back against your heels, and let your upper body rest gently on your thighs without diminishing the contact between your heels and your bottom. Extend the arms as far forward as you can. The head is always an extension of the spine.

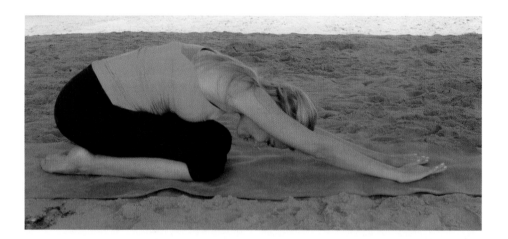

Biceps curls

Stand tall. Hold a weight (e.g., water bottle, backpack, purse) in each hand. Choose the same amount of weight for both hands. During this exercise, the upper arms and elbows rest against the ribcage and do not move. The wrists are always an extension of the spine. Now bend your elbows and move your hands toward your upper body until you feel the maximum amount of tension in your biceps. Then return your arms to an almost fully extended position.

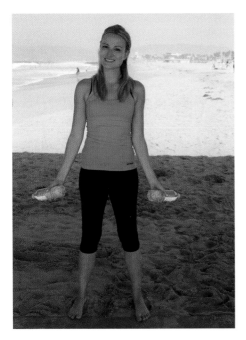
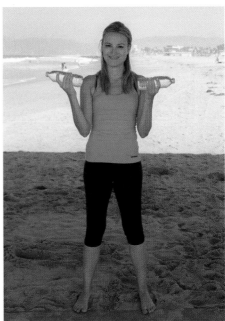

Lateral raise

Stand tall. Hold a weight (e.g., water bottle, backpack, purse) in each hand. Choose the same amount of weight for both hands. During this exercise, the arms are extended and never bend. Now raise your arms to the sides until the elbows are at forehead-level, and then slowly lower them to the starting position.

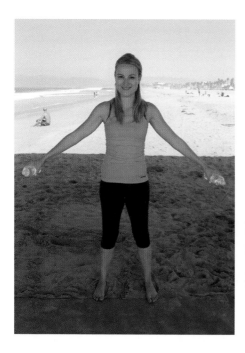 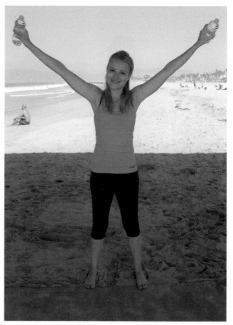

Shoulder press

Stand tall. Hold a weight (e.g., water bottle, backpack, purse) in each hand. Choose the same amount of weight for both hands. Now raise your arms to the sides until your upper arms are parallel to the ground. Your forearms are in a vertical position. Now extend your arms with the weights up until they are nearly straight. Then reverse the motion until your upper arms are once again parallel to the ground.

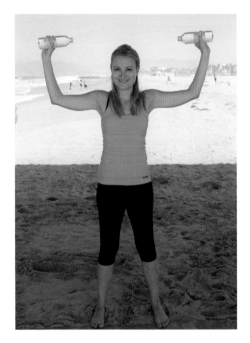 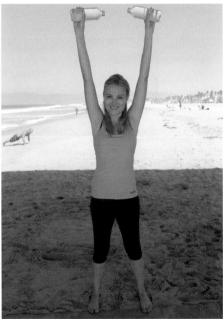

Triceps press

Slightly bend your knees. Now bend the upper body forward. During this exercise, the upper arms remain in contact with the ribcage. Now extend your arms along with the weights from the bent position to an extended position. Try to achieve maximum extension. The head is always an extension of the spine.

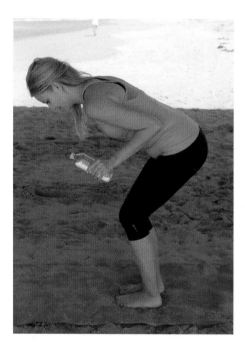 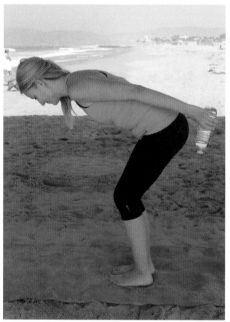

Cat-cow

Get on all fours. Movements performed in this position are slow and controlled. First round your back as much as possible into the cat position; immediately after, arch your back into the cow position.

Important: These movements must be slow and controlled. Avoid fast, jerky movements.

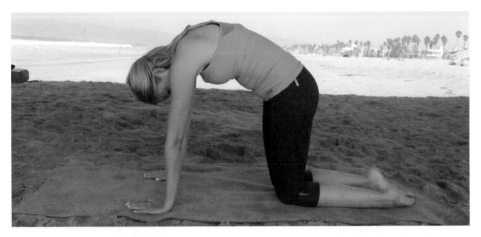

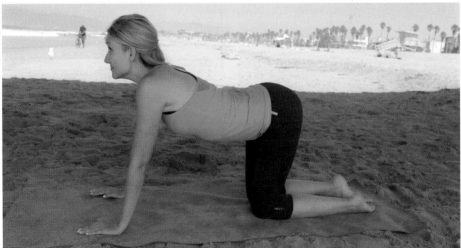

6.2   LEGS AND BUTT

Left-right leaps

First set up a small obstacle. You can use a rolled up towel, a bottle, or just a t-shirt. Now leap over the obstacle with one leg. Take off with the right leg and land on the left leg, and vice-versa. Try to increase the tempo and jump high.

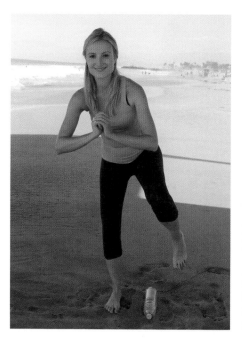 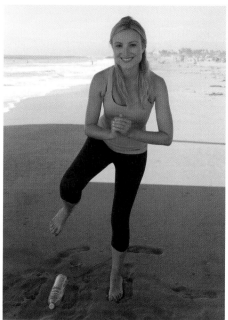

Wall sit

Stand with your back against a wall. Slide your back down the wall until there is a 90-degree angle between the upper and lower legs. Hold this position for the specified amount of time. As you do so, try to keep the bulk of your weight on your heels.

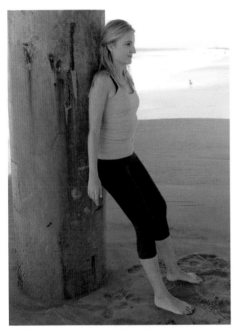 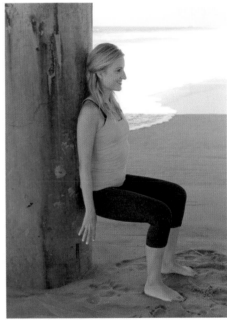

Squats

Stand with your feet slightly wider than hip-width apart and toes pointing forward. The bulk of your weight is on your heels and there is little weight on your toes. Now lower your bottom and try to get as low as you can while keeping the upper body as straight as possible.

Important: Don't let your knees come forward. The kneecap should never be in front of the big toe.

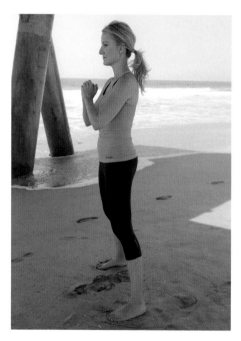 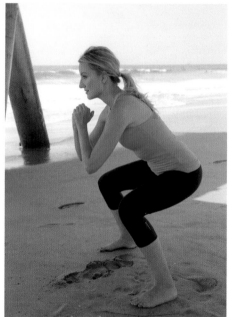

Cross-legged squat

Stand with your legs crossed and toes pointing forward. The upper body is straight, the bulk of your weight is on the front heel, and there is very little weight on your toes. Now the back knee bends toward the ground while the upper body remains straight. The lower the position, the more intense the exercise.

Important: Work both sides!

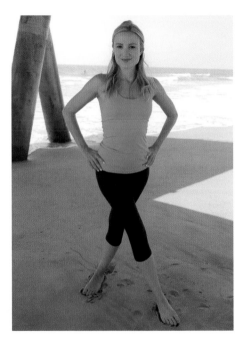
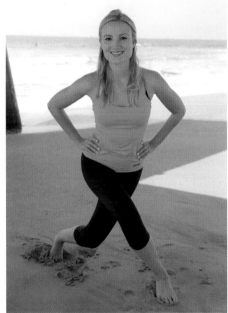

Toe squats

Stand with your feet slightly wider than hip-width apart. Now balance on your toes. Staying on your toes, perform a squat. Try NOT to shift your weight forward but keep your body as vertical as possible as you lower down into the squat. The lower the better. The upper body stays straight and the head is an extension of the spine.

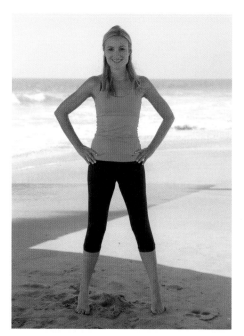 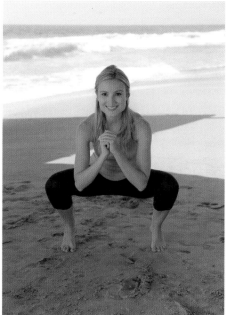

Squat + side kick

Begin by standing with your feet slightly wider than hip-width apart and your toes pointing forward. The bulk of your weight is on your heels with very little weight on your toes. Now lower your bottom as much as you can while keeping the upper body straight. Return to the starting position, and in one fluid motion, perform a side kick. Alternate sides. As you do so, try to kick as high as you can. Immediately after, return to the deep final position without interruption.

Important: Don't let the knees slide forward. The kneecap should never be in front of the big toe.

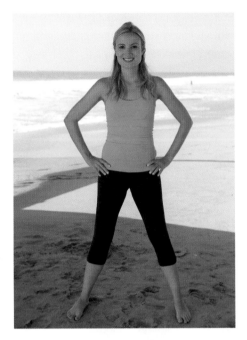

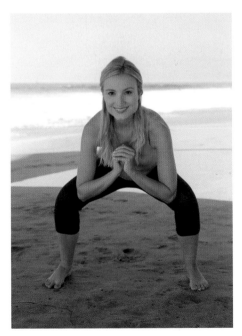

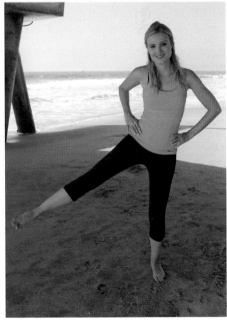

Plié squats

Start with your feet shoulder-width apart. Turn your toes out as far as you can. The upper body remains straight during the entire exercise and the head is an extension of the spine. Now lower your hips as much as you can and then return to the starting position.

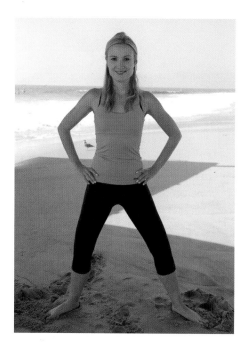 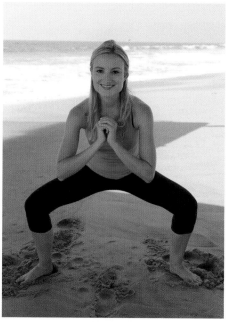

Single-leg squat

Begin by standing on one leg. Stand up straight and steady. Now bend the supporting leg to get into a deep squat. As you do so, make sure that your weight is primarily on your front heel and that the knee of the supporting leg does not slide forward.

Important: Work both sides!

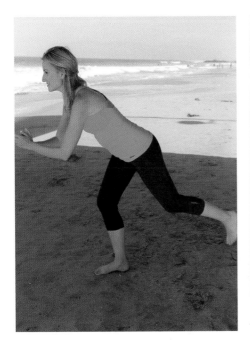 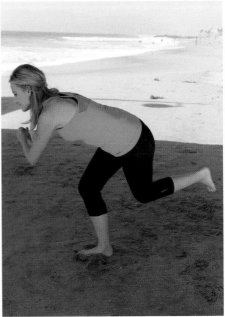

Side lunge

Begin by standing in a slight straddle position. Now shift your weight to one side with a straight upper body while keeping the bulk of your weight on the heel of the leg you shifted your weight to. Toes point forward.

Important: Work both sides!

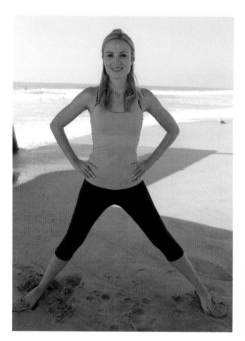 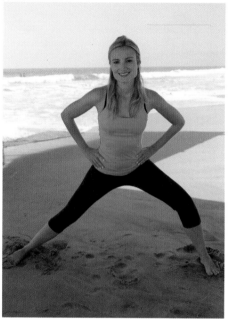

Forward lunge

Step into a forward lunge. Toes always point forward, the upper body is straight, and the bulk of your upper-body weight is always on the front heel. There is no weight on the toes during the entire exercise. Now drop the back knee as low as possible without shifting your weight forward.

Important: Work both sides!

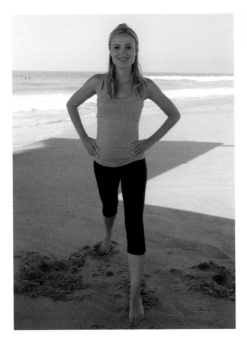
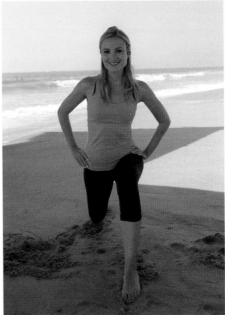

Lunge + rotation

Step into a forward lunge. Toes always point forward, the upper body is straight, and the bulk of your upper-body weight is always on the front heel. There is no weight on the toes during the entire exercise. Now drop the back knee as low as you can without shifting your weight forward. Finally, rotate the upper body toward the front knee. For instance, if your right knee is in front, rotate your upper body as far to the right as you can. The goal is to achieve maximum mobility and range of motion with the upper body.

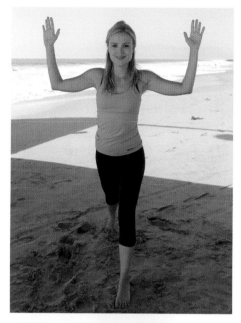

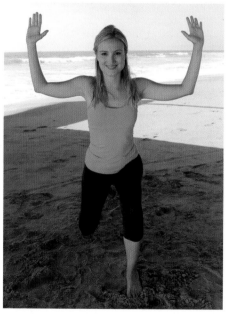

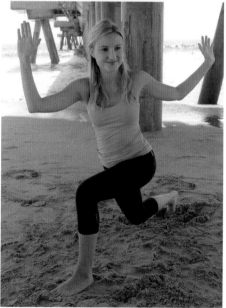

Two-legged heel raises

Stand firm with your feet hip-width apart. Now raise your heels as high as you can, balancing on your toes. Both legs are straight and all of the movement takes place in the ankle joint.

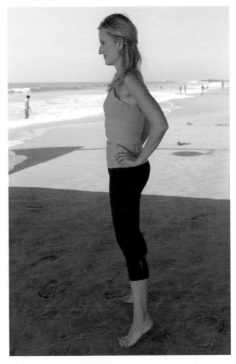

One-legged heel raises

Stand firmly on one leg. Now raise the heel of your supporting leg as high as you can. The supporting leg is always straight and all the movement takes place in the ankle joint.

Important: Work both sides!

 If you have balance problems, you can start by holding on to a wall.

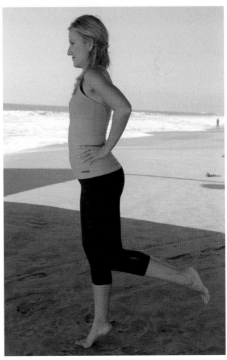

90-degree back kick

Begin by getting on all fours. Form a 90-degree angle from thigh to calf with both legs. Maintain this right angle during the entire exercise. Now move one leg back and up to achieve maximum extension. Immediately return to the starting position, but do not allow the knee to touch the ground.

Important: *Work both sides!*

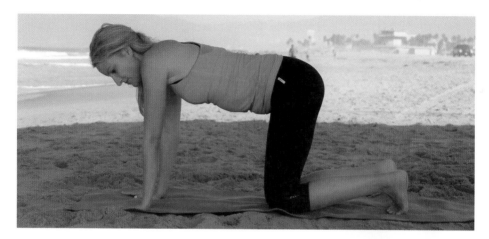

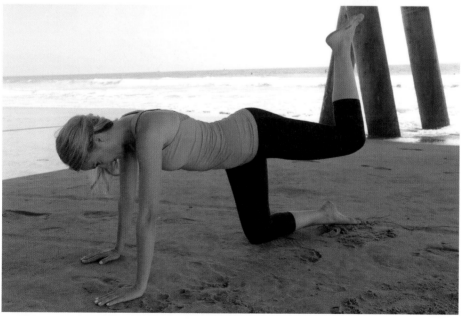

Extended back kick

Start on all fours. From this position, extend one leg straight back and up as far as you can. Then return to the starting position and perform another repetition according to the instructions.

Important: Work both sides!

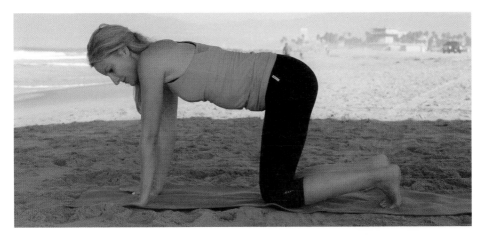

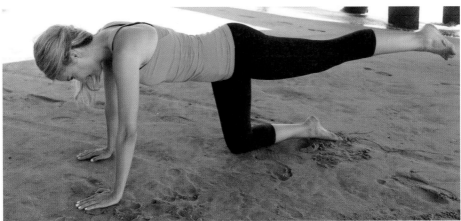

90-degree two-point back kick

Begin on all fours. From this position, form a 90-degree angle from thigh to calf with both legs. Place one hand on the opposite shoulder. Now lift one leg as high as you can, trying to achieve maximum extension. Immediately after, return to the starting position, but don't let the knee touch the ground.

Important: Work both sides!

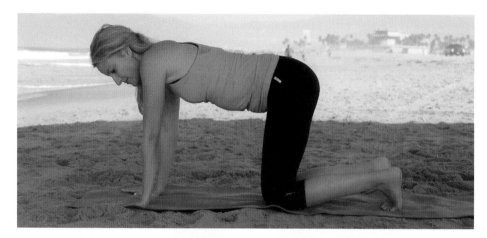

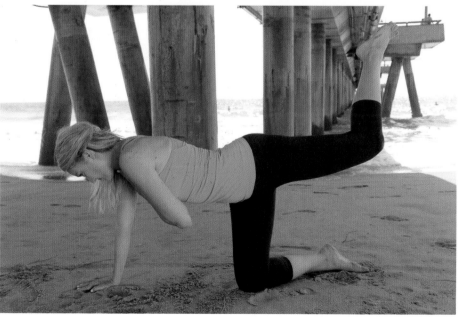

Kneeling hip opener

Start on all fours. In this position, keep your upper body as steady as possible as you perform a 90-degree lateral rise with one leg. The goal is to laterally raise the knee as high as possible. Immediately after, return to the starting position and then perform another repetition as instructed.

Important: Work both sides!

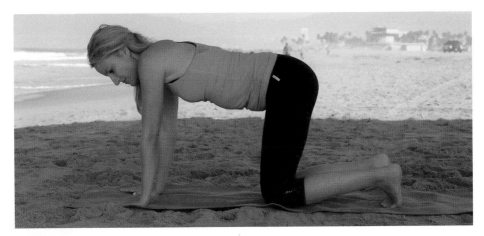

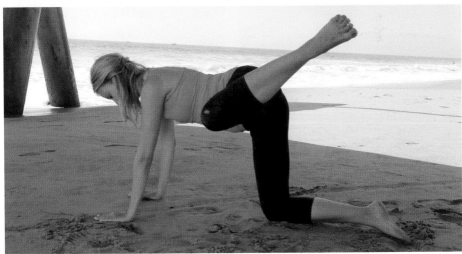

Standing hip abduction

Stand tall in your starting position. Next raise one extended leg to the side as high as you can WITHOUT moving your upper body. Make sure only the leg moves.

Important: *Work both sides!*

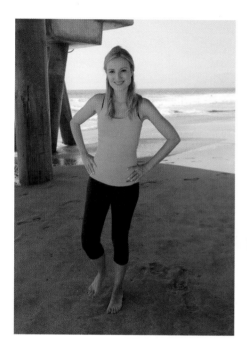 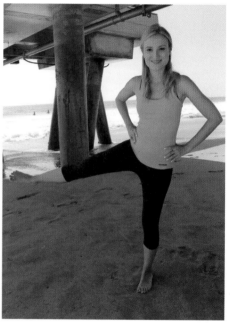

Back leg lift

Stand firm. Support yourself with your hands against a wall, and after that do not change your body position, only the fully extended leg performing the back lift moves.

Important: Switch sides and always try to create maximum tension in your gluteal muscles.

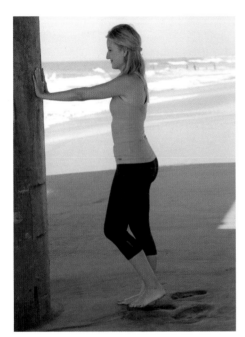 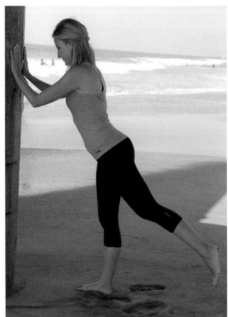

Standing adduction

Stand firmly with your feet hip-width apart. Now move one leg across the other leg as far as possible.

Important: *Work both sides!*

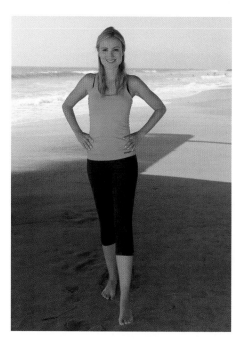 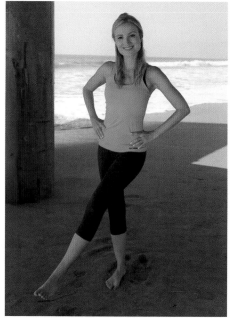

Standing scale

Stand on one leg. Now move your upper body forward and down while extending one leg as far back and up as possible. The goal is to position the upper body and the extended leg in a horizontal position. The supporting knee is slightly bent.

Important: Work both sides!

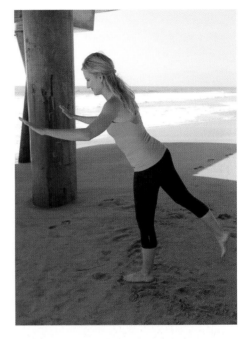

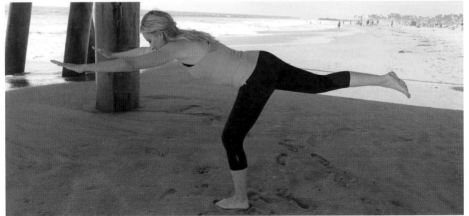

Bridge + leg extension

Lie on your back with your knees bent and make sure that your legs are parallel. Now move your heels close to your bottom and extend one leg upward. Next, raise your hips as high as you can while making sure your hips don't tilt left or right, but remain straight.

Important: Work both sides!

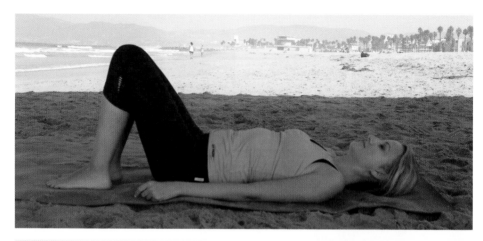

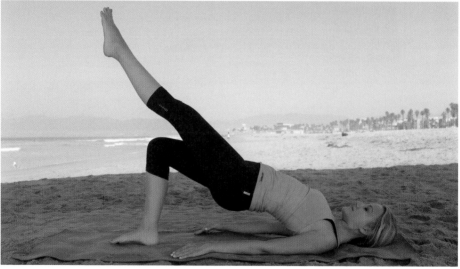

Prone position + diagonal extension

Lie on your stomach in a straight position; the head is an extension of the spine. Rest your forehead on the ground. Now raise one extended leg and the opposite extended arm as high as you can.

Important: Work both sides!

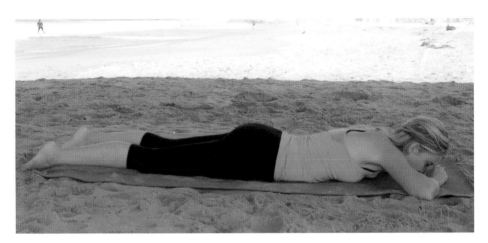

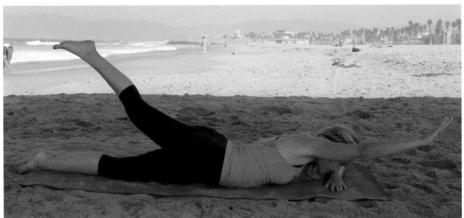

Prone position + hip extension

Lie on your stomach. Extend your legs so they are parallel. During this exercise, the upper body stays relaxed and does not move. Raise both legs off the ground as high as you can, actively tighten your gluteal muscles, and open your legs as wide as you can. Then return to the starting position. As you do so, don't let your legs come all the way down but return to the final position.

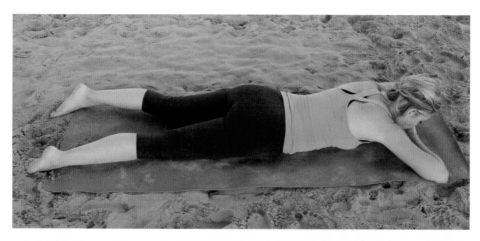

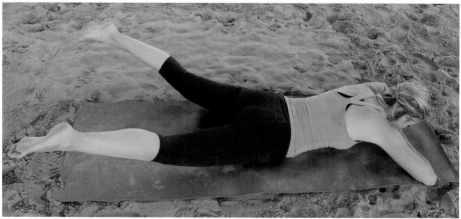

Side abduction

Lie on your side and extend your body as much as possible. Raise the upper leg as high as you can. As you do so, make sure only the leg moves and the upper body remains still.

Important: *Work both sides!*

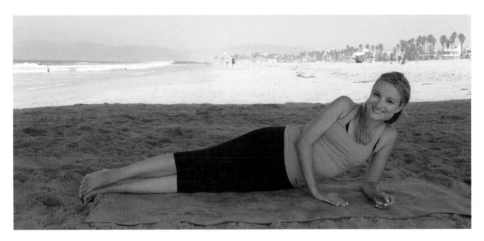

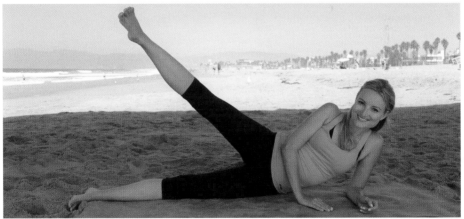

Side adduction

Lie on your side. Bend the top knee and plant the foot on the ground. The bottom leg remains extended and the upper body is in a stable position. Now lift the bottom leg as high as you can. Avoid any upper-body movement.

Important: Work both sides!

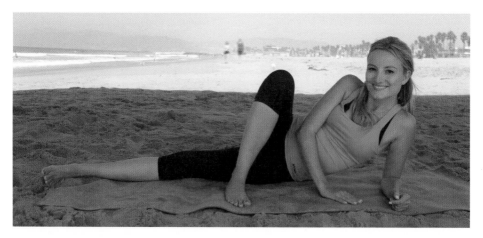

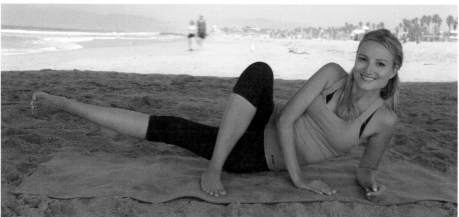

Crossover reach

Stand in a straddle position. Legs are straight and arms are fully extended. Bend forward and reach with your right hand toward your left toe, and then with your left hand toward your right toe.

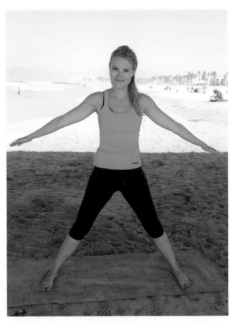

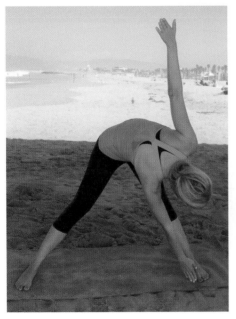

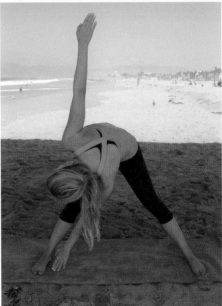

Seated back stretch

In a seated position, extend your legs in a parallel position and straighten your knees as much as possible. In the starting position, the upper body is already slightly bent forward. Now extend your arms forward and try to reach your toes with your hands.

Important: Keep your feet flexed during this exercise.

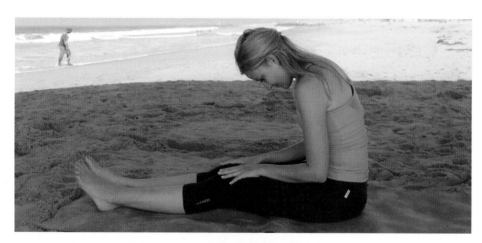

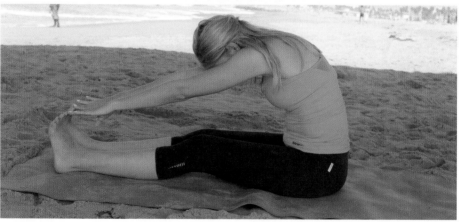

Cobbler's stretch

Start in a seated position. Now bring the soles of your feet together and move your heels closer to the body. Drop your knees as close to the ground as possible to deepen the stretch. Roll the upper body forward slightly.

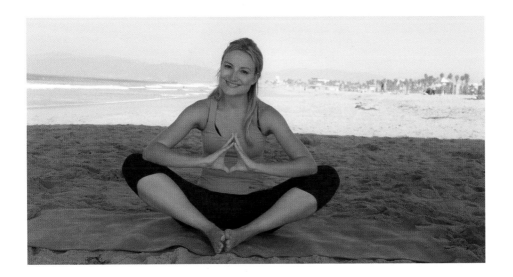

Hand-to-foot stretch

Start in a push-up position. Raise your hips as high as you can and push your heels toward the ground. Legs are straight. Now move your toes closer to your hands by making tiny steps.

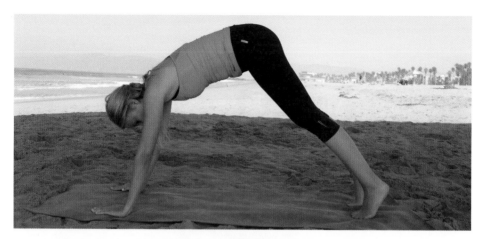

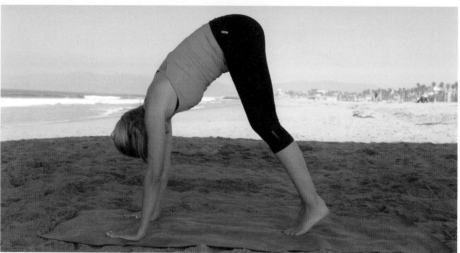

Quadriceps stretch

Stand tall. Now pull one heel toward your bottom. Keep your upper body as straight as possible.

Important: Stretch both sides!

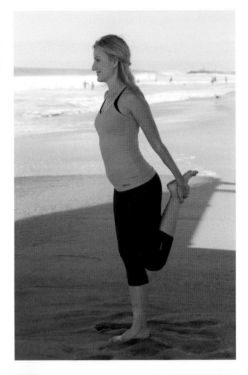

Calf stretch

Get in a lunge position. Place both hands against a wall. Shift your weight as far forward as you can while pushing the back heel toward the ground, so you can feel a stretch in the calf.

Important: Stretch both sides!

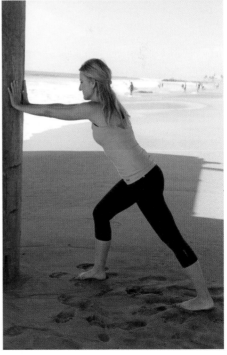

Cross-legged gluteal stretch

Stand firmly on one leg. Now grip the heel and calf of the free leg with both hands and move the leg into the highest possible final position.

Important: Stretch both sides!

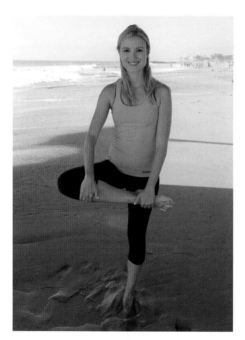 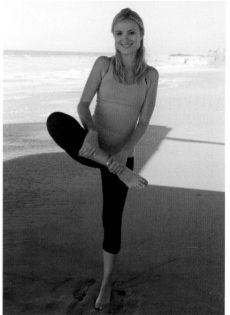

Side quadriceps stretch

Lie on your side. Now bend the knee of the upper leg to move your heel toward your bottom. Gripping the ankle, pull that thigh back as far as you can. Now actively push the upper hip forward to deepen the stretch.

Important: Stretch both sides!

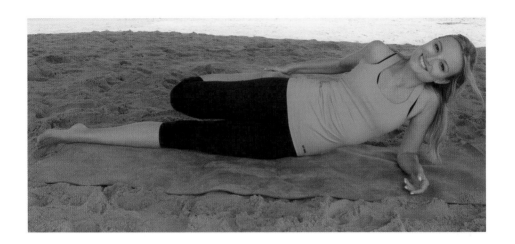

Kneeling hip opener

To start this stretch, step into a classic forward lunge and rest the back knee on the ground. Now create a 90-degree angle between the front calf and thigh. Do the same between the back calf and thigh. Extend the arms overhead. Now actively push the open hip forward, and slowly and carefully arch your back so the frontal muscle chain is really extended.

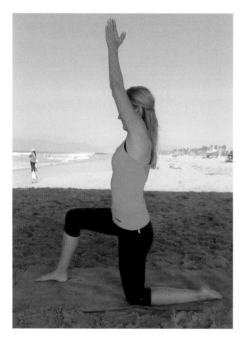 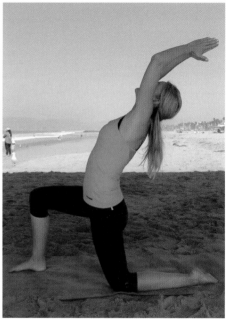

Seated cross-legged gluteal stretch

Start in an upright seated position with your legs extended forward. Now bend the right knee and plant the right foot to the inside of the left thigh. Turn your upper body to the right so you can rest the left upper arm or elbow against the outside of the right leg at knee level. Now press the right knee to the left until you feel a stretch at the outside of the thigh, primarily in the gluteal area.

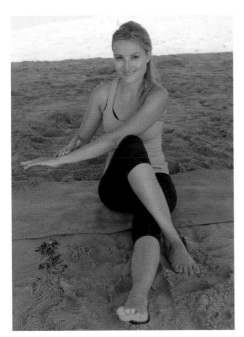 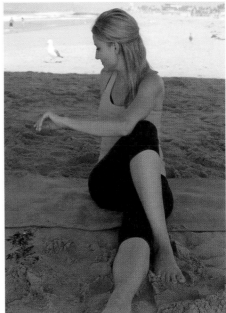

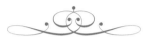

7 WORKOUT

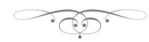

7 Workout

Important: The workout is based on time and not the number of repetitions. It is therefore essential that you adhere to the speed of movement and have a timer on hand. The respective performance level determines the length of your workout.

CLASSIFICATION:

Performance level 1

Has never exercised, has not exercised in a long time, exercises less then 1 hour per week.

Suggested BREAK LENGTH: 30 seconds

Performance level 2

Exercises occasionally, 1-3 hours per week max.

Suggested BREAK LENGTH: 20 seconds

Performance level 3

Exercises regularly, 3 hours or more per week

Suggested BREAK LENGTH: 15 seconds

Warm-up: Complete each exercise once as a warm-up. IMPORTANT: The warm-up can only take half the time of the actual set. Example: If the specified set duration is 40 seconds for one exercise, the warm-up is only 20 seconds.

PLEASE NOTE: If you feel pain during an exercise, you can of course switch the exercise with a different one of your choosing from the exercise catalog (chapter 6), but this should be an exception rather than the norm.

HOW do I work out by time? You have a timer in front of you. You also have the specified set duration as well as the speed of movement. Please always observe all parameters. If you have not completely finished an exercise but the specified set duration has been met, you can break off the exercise and continue with the next exercise.

Whenever you do static exercises, hold the position unchanged for the specified set duration.

WEEK 1:

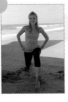
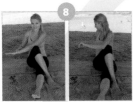
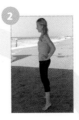
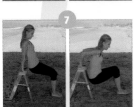
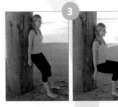

Performance level 1

Number of sets: 2-3

Set break: 30 seconds (or less)

Warm-up: half a set of each exercise
serves as the warm-up

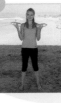
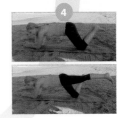
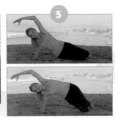
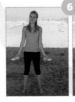

Exercise frequency: 3x per week + one day break in between workouts

Speed of movement: 3-1-3 seconds: That means 3 seconds from the starting position to the final position. Hold the final position for 1 second, and then return to the starting position within 3 seconds.

Set duration: 40 seconds per exercise (i.e., you will need approximately 9 minutes for a circuit of 8 exercises, and a maximum of 30 minutes for 2-3 sets).

Workout:
1. Forward lunge, pg. 107
2. Heel raises, both legs, pg. 109
3. Wall sit, pg. 99
4. Kneeling forearm plank + leg extension, pg. 54
5. Kneeling forearm side plank, pg. 64
6. Biceps curls, pg. 93
7. 90-degree dips, pg. 48
8. Seated cross-legged gluteal stretch, pg. 131

WEEK 2:

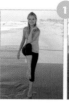

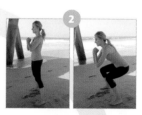

Performance level 1

Number of sets: 2-3

Set break: 30 seconds (or less)

Warm-up: half a set of each exercise serves as the warm-up

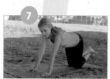
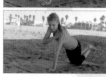
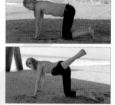
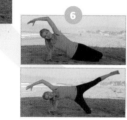
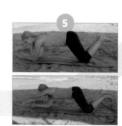

Exercise frequency: 3x per week + one day break in between workouts

Speed of movement: 3-1-3 seconds: That means 3 seconds from the starting position to the final position. Hold the final position for 1 second, and then return to the starting position within 3 seconds.

Set duration: 45 seconds per exercise

Workout:
1. Standing crunch, pg. 41
2. Squats, pg. 100
3. Forward lunge, pg. 107
4. Kneeling hip opener, pg. 113
5. Kneeling forearm plank + arm extension, pg. 56
6. Kneeling forearm side plank + leg extension, pg. 65
7. Kneeling shoulder tap, pg. 76
8. Cobbler's stretch, pg. 125

WEEK 3:

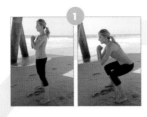

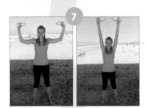

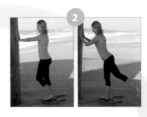

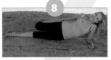

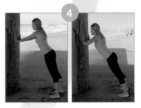

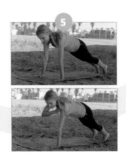

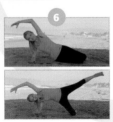

Performance level 1

Number of sets: 2-3
Set break: 30 seconds (or less)
Warm-up: half a set of each exercise
serves as the warm-up

Exercise frequency: 3-4x per week

Speed of movement: 3-1-3 seconds: That means 3 seconds from the starting position to the final position. Hold the final position for 1 second, and then return to the starting position within 3 seconds.

Set duration: 50 seconds per exercise

Workout:
1. Squats, pg. 100
2. Back leg lift, pg. 115
3. Standing adduction, pg. 116
4. 45° push-ups, pg. 42
5. Shoulder tap, pg. 77
6. Kneeling forearm side plank + leg extension, pg. 65
7. Shoulder press, pg. 95
8. Gluteal stretch, pg. 129

WEEK 4:

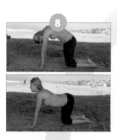

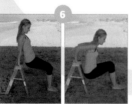
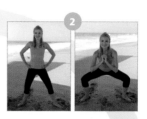
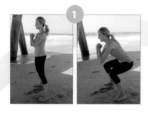
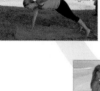
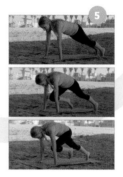
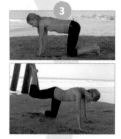
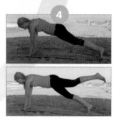

Performance level 1

Number of sets: 2-3

Set break: 30 seconds (or less)

Warm-up: half a set of each exercise serves as the warm-up

Exercise frequency: 3-4x per week

Speed of movement: 3-1-3 seconds: That means 3 seconds from the starting position to the final position. Hold the final position for 1 second, and then return to the starting position within 3 seconds.

Set duration: 55 seconds per exercise

Workout:
1. Squats, pg. 100
2. Plié squats, pg. 104
3. 90° back kick, pg. 110
4. Full plank + leg extension, pg. 61
5. Mountain climber, pg. 78
6. 90-degree dips, pg. 48
7. Push-up position + lateral extension, pg. 49
8. Cat-cow, pg. 97

WEEK 5:

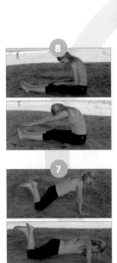
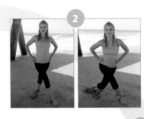

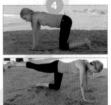
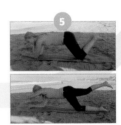
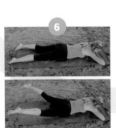
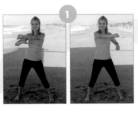

Performance level 1

Number of sets: 2-3
Set break: 30 seconds (or less)
Warm-up: half a set of each exercise serves as the warm-up

Exercise frequency: 3-4x per week

Speed of movement: 2-1-2 seconds: That means 2 seconds from the starting position to the final position. Hold the final position for 1 second, and then return to the starting position within 2 seconds.

Set duration: 55 seconds per exercise

Workout:
1. Shadowboxing, pg. 40
2. Cross-legged squat, pg. 101
3. Plié squats, pg. 104
4. Straight back kick, pg. 111
5. Kneeling forearm plank + diagonal extension, pg. 55
6. Prone position + hip extension, pg. 120
7. Kneeling push-ups, pg. 44
8. Seated back stretch, pg. 124

WEEK 6:

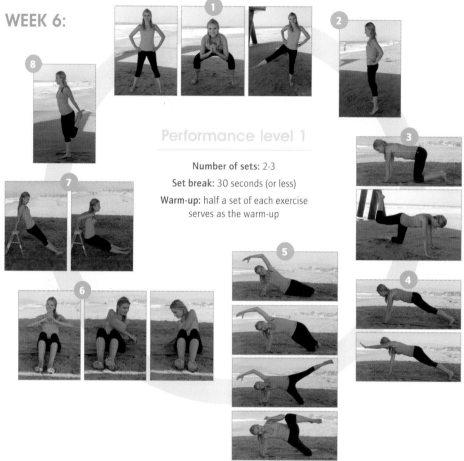

Performance level 1

Number of sets: 2-3

Set break: 30 seconds (or less)

Warm-up: half a set of each exercise serves as the warm-up

Exercise frequency: 4x per week

Speed of movement: 2-1-2 seconds: That means 2 seconds from the starting position to the final position. Hold the final position for 1 second, and then return to the starting position within 2 seconds.

Set duration: 45 seconds per exercise

Workout:
1. Squat + side kick, pg. 103
2. Two-legged heel-raises, pg. 109
3. 90-degree back kick, pg. 110
4. Full plank + arm extension, pg. 62
5. Kneeling forearm side plank + crunch, pg. 66
6. Seated crunch, pg. 84
7. Extended dips, pg. 51
8. Quadriceps stretch, pg. 127

WEEK 7: *CORE WEEK*

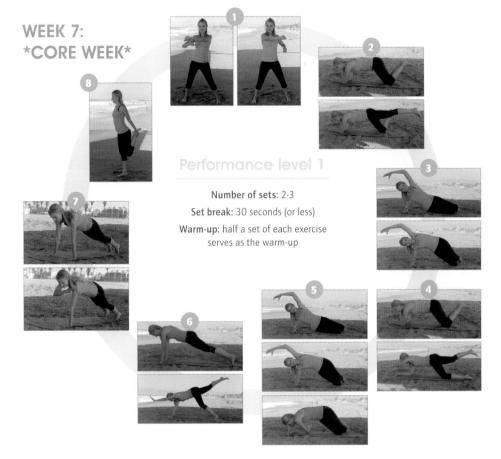

Performance level 1

Number of sets: 2-3

Set break: 30 seconds (or less)

Warm-up: half a set of each exercise serves as the warm-up

Exercise frequency: 4x per week

Speed of movement: 2-1-2 seconds: That means 2 seconds from the starting position to the final position. Hold the final position for 1 second, and then return to the starting position within 2 seconds.

Set duration: 45 seconds per exercise

Workout:
1. Shadowboxing, pg. 40
2. Kneeling forearm plank + leg extension, pg. 54
3. Kneeling forearm side plank, pg. 64
4. Kneeling forearm plank + diagonal extension, pg. 55
5. Kneeling forearm side plank + twist, pg. 68
6. Full plank + diagonal extension, pg. 63
7. Shoulder tap, pg. 77
8. Quadriceps stretch, pg. 127

WEEK 8: *TIGHT BUNS WEEK*

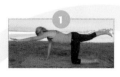
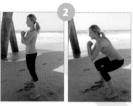
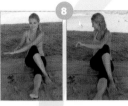
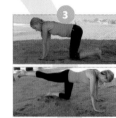
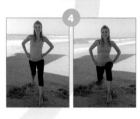
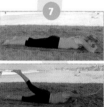
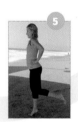

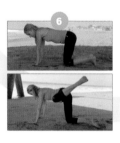
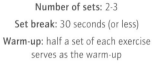

Performance level 1

Number of sets: 2-3
Set break: 30 seconds (or less)
Warm-up: half a set of each exercise serves as the warm-up

Exercise frequency: 4x per week

Speed of movement: 2-1-2 seconds: That means 2 seconds from the starting position to the final position. Hold the final position for 1 second, and then return to the starting position within 2 seconds.

Set duration: 55 seconds per exercise

Workout:
1. All-fours position + diagonal extension, pg. 87
2. Squats, pg. 100
3. Straight back kick, pg. 111
4. Forward lunge, pg. 107
5. One-legged heel raises, pg. 109
6. Kneeling hip opener, pg. 113
7. Prone position + and diagonal extension, pg. 119
8. Seated cross-legged gluteal stretch, pg. 131

WEEK 9:
PHASE I FINAL

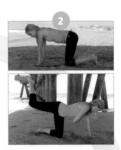
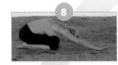
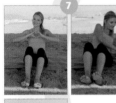
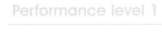
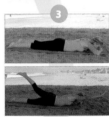
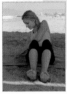
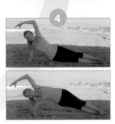
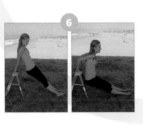
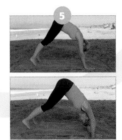

Performance level 1

Number of sets: 2-3

Set break: 30 seconds (or less)

Warm-up: half a set of each exercise
serves as the warm-up

Exercise frequency: 4x per week

Speed of movement: Super slow! 4-1-4 seconds: That means 4 seconds from the starting position to the final position. Hold the final position for 1 second, and then return to the starting position within 4 seconds.

Set duration: 60 seconds per exercise

Workout:
1. Left-right leaps, pg. 98
2. 90-degree two-point back kick, pg. 112
3. Prone position + diagonal extension, pg. 119
4. Extended forearm side plank, pg. 70
5. Parachutist push-ups, pg. 50
6. Extended dips, pg. 51
7. Seated crunch, pg. 84
8. Child's pose, pg. 92

143

WEEK 10: PHASE II FINAL

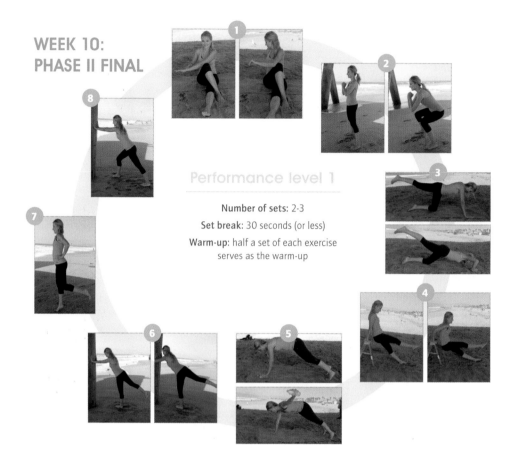

Performance level 1

Number of sets: 2-3
Set break: 30 seconds (or less)
Warm-up: half a set of each exercise serves as the warm-up

Exercise frequency: 4x per week

Speed of movement: Super slow! 4-1-4 seconds: That means 4 seconds from the starting position to the final position. Hold the final position for 1 second, and then return to the starting position within 4 seconds.

Set duration: 60 seconds per exercise

Workout:
1. Seated cross-legged gluteal stretch, pg. 131
2. Squats, pg. 100
3. Kneeling three-point push-ups, pg. 45
4. Three-point dips, pg. 52
5. Push-up position + lateral extension, pg. 49
6. 45-degree three-point push-ups, pg. 43
7. Two-legged heel raises, pg. 109
8. Calf stretch, pg. 127

WEEK 1:

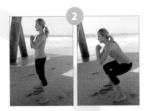
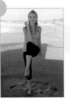

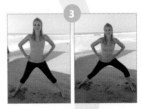

Performance level 2

Number of sets: 2-3

Set break: 20 seconds (or less)

Warm-up: half a set of each exercise serves as the warm-up

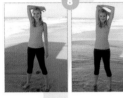
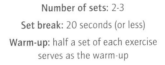
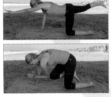
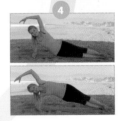
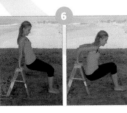
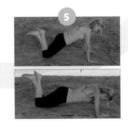

Exercise frequency: 3x per week

Speed of movement: 2-1-2 seconds: That means 2 seconds from the starting position to the final position. Hold the final position for 1 second, and then return to the starting position within 2 seconds.

Set duration: 55 seconds per exercise

Workout:
1. Standing crunch, pg. 41
2. Squats, pg. 100
3. Side lunge, pg. 106
4. Extended forearm side plank, pg. 70
5. Kneeling push-ups, pg. 44
6. 90-degree dips, pg. 48
7. Diagonal all-fours position + crunch, pg. 88
8. Triceps stretch, pg. 89

WEEK 2:

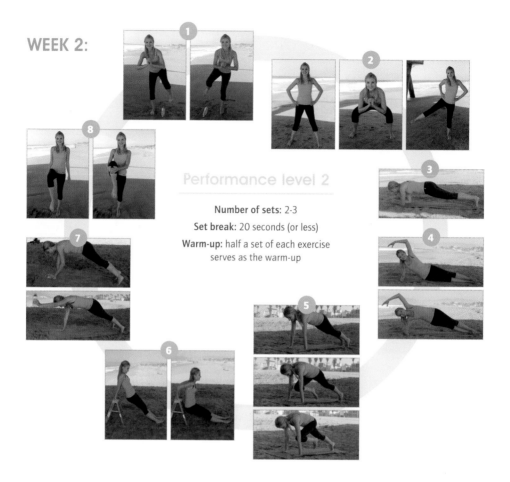

Performance level 2

Number of sets: 2-3

Set break: 20 seconds (or less)

Warm-up: half a set of each exercise serves as the warm-up

Exercise frequency: 3x per week

Speed of movement: 2-1-2 seconds: That means 2 seconds from the starting position to the final position. Hold the final position for 1 second, and then return to the starting position within 2 seconds.

Set duration: 55 seconds per exercise

Workout:
1. Left-right leaps, pg. 98
2. Squat + side kick, pg. 103
3. Forearm plank, pg. 57
4. Extended forearm side plank, pg. 70
5. Mountain climber, pg. 78
6. Extended dips, pg. 51
7. Push-up position + forward extension, pg. 47
8. Gluteal stretch, pg. 91

WEEK 3:

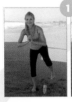
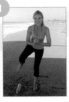
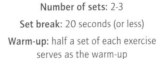
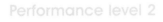
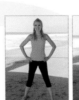
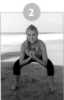

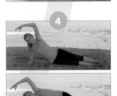
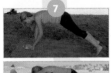
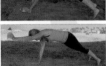
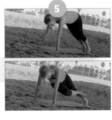

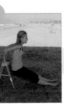
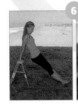

Performance level 2

Number of sets: 2-3

Set break: 20 seconds (or less)

Warm-up: half a set of each exercise serves as the warm-up

Exercise frequency: 3-4x per week

Speed of movement: 2-1-2 seconds: That means 2 seconds from the starting position to the final position. Hold the final position for 1 second, and then return to the starting position within 2 seconds.

Set duration: 55 seconds per exercise

Workout:
1. Left-right leaps, pg. 98
2. Squat + side kick, pg. 103
3. Forearm plank + leg extension, pg. 58
4. Extended forearm side plank, pg. 70
5. Diagonal mountain climber, pg. 80
6. Extended dips, pg. 51
7. Push-up position + forward extension, pg. 47
8. Cross-legged gluteal stretch, pg. 128

WEEK 4:

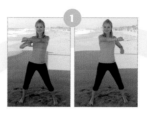

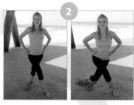

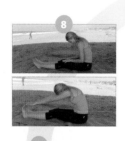

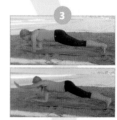

Performance level 2

Number of sets: 2-3
Set break: 20 seconds (or less)
Warm-up: half a set of each exercise serves as the warm-up

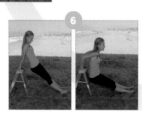

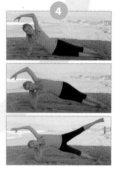

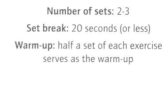

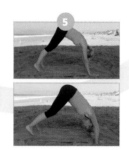

Exercise frequency: 3-4x per week

Speed of movement: 2-1-2 seconds: That means 2 seconds from the starting position to the final position. Hold the final position for 1 second, and then return to the starting position within 2 seconds.

Set duration: 55 seconds per exercise

Workout:
1. Shadowboxing, pg. 40
2. Cross-legged squat, pg. 101
3. Forearm plank + arm extension, pg. 59
4. Extended forearm side plank + leg raise, pg. 71
5. Parachutist push-ups, pg. 50
6. Extended dips, pg. 51
7. Push-up position + lateral extension, pg. 49
8. Seated back stretch, pg. 124

WEEK 5:

Performance level 2

Number of sets: 2-3

Set break: 20 seconds (or less)

Warm-up: half a set of each exercise serves as the warm-up

Exercise frequency: 3-4x per week

Speed of movement: 2-1-2 seconds: That means 2 seconds from the starting position to the final position. Hold the final position for 1 second, and then return to the starting position within 2 seconds.

Set duration: 55 seconds per exercise

Workout:
1. Wall sit, pg. 99
2. Plié squats, pg. 104
3. Forearm plank + leg extension, pg. 58
4. Extended forearm side plank + twist, pg. 72
5. Biceps curls, pg. 93
6. Shoulder press, pg. 95
7. Lateral raise, pg. 94
8. Triceps stretch, pg. 89

WEEK 6:

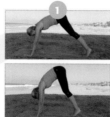
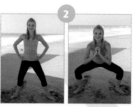
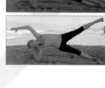
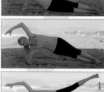
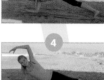
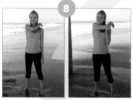
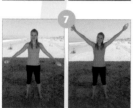
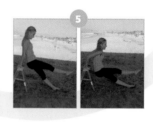
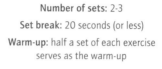
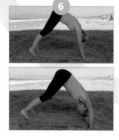

Performance level 2

Number of sets: 2-3

Set break: 20 seconds (or less)

Warm-up: half a set of each exercise serves as the warm-up

Exercise frequency: 4x per week

Speed of movement: 2-1-2 seconds: That means 2 seconds from the starting position to the final position. Hold the final position for 1 second, and then return to the starting position within 2 seconds.

Set duration: 60 seconds per exercise

Workout:
1. Hand-to-foot stretch, pg. 126
2. Plié squats, pg. 104
3. Forearm plank + diagonal extension, pg. 60
4. Extended forearm side plank + leg raise, pg. 71
5. Three-point dips, pg. 52
6. Parachutist push-ups, pg. 50
7. Lateral raise, pg. 94
8. Shoulder stretch pg. 90

WEEK 7: *CORE WEEK*

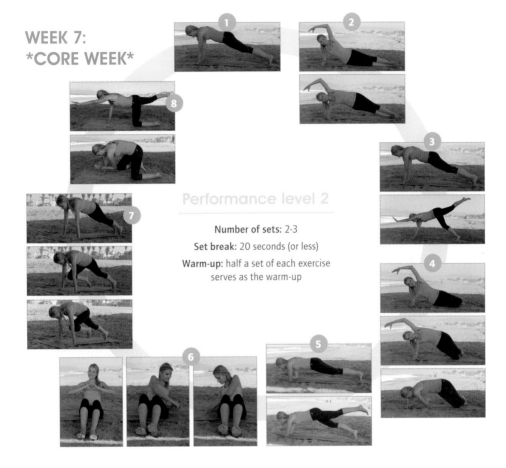

Performance level 2

Number of sets: 2-3

Set break: 20 seconds (or less)

Warm-up: half a set of each exercise serves as the warm-up

Exercise frequency: 4x per week

Speed of movement: 2-1-2 seconds: That means 2 seconds from the starting position to the final position. Hold the final position for 1 second, and then return to the starting position within 2 seconds.

Set duration: 60 seconds per exercise

Workout:
1. Full plank, pg. 60
2. Extended forearm side plank, pg. 70
3. Full plank + diagonal extension, pg. 63
4. Kneeling forearm side plank + twist, pg. 68
5. Forearm plank + leg extension, pg. 58
6. Seated crunch, pg. 84
7. Mountain climber, pg. 78
8. Diagonal all-fours position + crunch, pg. 88

WEEK 8: *TIGHT BUNS WEEK*

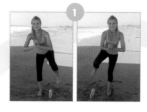
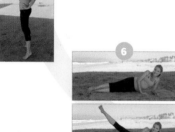
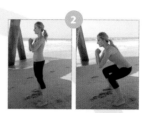
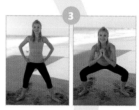
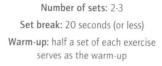
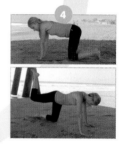
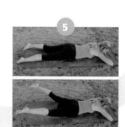
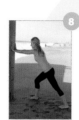

Performance level 2

Number of sets: 2-3
Set break: 20 seconds (or less)
Warm-up: half a set of each exercise serves as the warm-up

Exercise frequency: 4x per week

Speed of movement: 2-1-2 seconds: That means 2 seconds from the starting position to the final position. Hold the final position for 1 second, and then return to the starting position within 2 seconds.

Set duration: 60 seconds per exercise

Workout:
1. Left-right leaps, pg. 98
2. Squats, pg. 100
3. Plié squats, pg. 104
4. 90-degree back kick, pg. 110
5. Prone position + hip extension, pg. 120
6. Side abduction, pg. 121
7. Two-legged heel raises, pg. 109
8. Calf stretch, pg. 127

WEEK 9: FINAL PHASE I

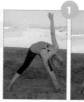

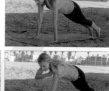
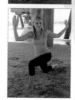

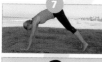

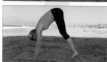

Performance level 2

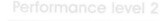

Number of sets: 2-3
Set break: 20 seconds (or less)
Warm-up: half a set of each exercise serves as the warm-up

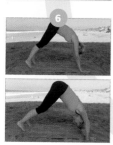

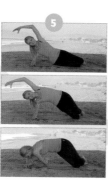

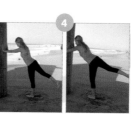

Exercise frequency: 4x per week

Speed of movement: 4-1-4 seconds: That means 4 seconds from the starting position to the final position. Hold the final position for 1 second, and then return to the starting position within 4 seconds.

Number of sets: 3

Set duration: 60 seconds per exercise

Workout:
1. Crossover reach, pg. 123
2. Lunge + rotation, pg. 108
3. Shoulder tap, pg. 77
4. 45-degree three-point push-ups, pg. 43
5. Kneeling forearm side plank + twist, pg. 68
6. Parachutist push-ups, pg. 50
7. Hand-to-foot stretch, pg. 126

WEEK 10:
FINAL PHASE II

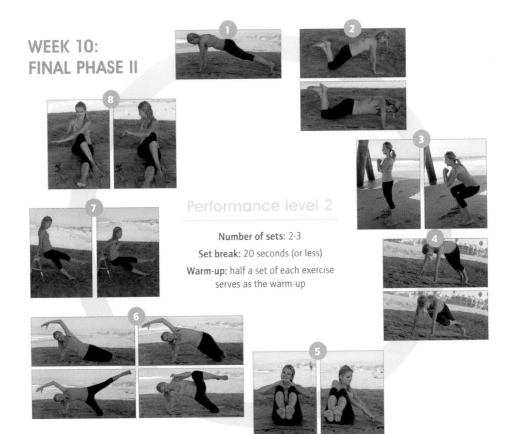

Performance level 2

Number of sets: 2-3

Set break: 20 seconds (or less)

Warm-up: half a set of each exercise serves as the warm-up

Exercise frequency: 4x per week

Speed of movement: 4-1-4 seconds: That means 4 seconds from the starting position to the final position. Hold the final position for 1 second, and then return to the starting position within 4 seconds.

Set duration: 60 seconds per exercise

Workout:
1. Forearm plank + diagonal extension, pg. 60
2. Kneeling push-ups, pg. 44
3. Squats, pg. 100
4. Diagonal mountain climber, pg. 80
5. Advanced seated crunch, pg. 85
6. Kneeling forearm side plank + crunch, pg. 66
7. Three-point dips, pg. 52
8. Seated cross-legged gluteal stretch, pg. 131

WEEK 1:

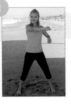
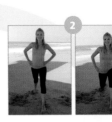
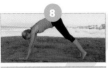
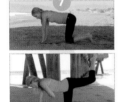
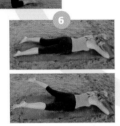
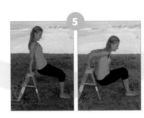
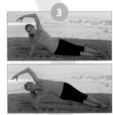
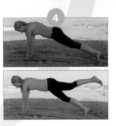
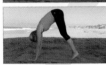

Performance level 3

Number of sets: 2-3

Set break: 10-15 seconds (or less)

Warm-up: half a set of each exercise
serves as the warm-up

Exercise frequency: 3x per week

Speed of movement: 2-1-2 seconds: That means 2 seconds from the starting position to the final position. Hold the final position for 1 second, and then return to the starting position within 2 seconds.

Set duration: 50 seconds per exercise

Workout:
1. Shadowboxing, pg. 40
2. Forward lunge, pg. 107
3. Extended forearm side plank, pg. 70
4. Full plank + leg extension, pg. 61
5. 90-degree dips, pg. 48
6. Prone position + hip extension, pg. 120
7. 90-degree two-point back kick, pg. 112
8. Hand-to-foot stretch, pg. 126

WEEK 2:

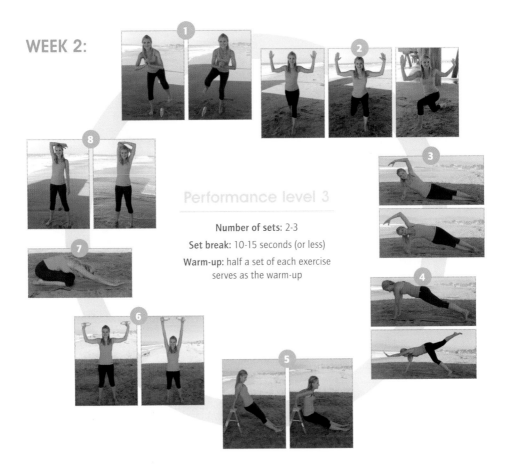

Performance level 3

Number of sets: 2-3
Set break: 10-15 seconds (or less)
Warm-up: half a set of each exercise
serves as the warm-up

Exercise frequency: 3-4x per week

Speed of movement: 2-1-2 seconds: That means 2 seconds from the starting position to the final position. Hold the final position for 1 second, and then return to the starting position within 2 seconds.

Set duration: 50 seconds per exercise

Workout:
1. Left-right leaps, pg. 98
2. Lunge + rotation, pg. 108
3. Extended forearm side plank, pg. 70
4. Full plank + diagonal extension, pg. 63
5. Extended dips, pg. 51
6. Shoulder press, pg. 95
7. Child's pose, pg. 92
8. Triceps stretch, pg. 89

WEEK 3:

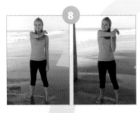

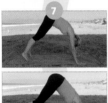

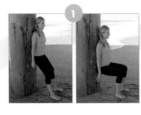

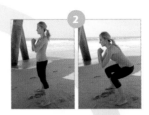

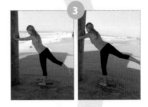

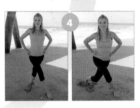

Performance level 3

Number of sets: 2-3
Set break: 10-15 seconds (or less)
Warm-up: half a set of each exercise
serves as the warm-up.

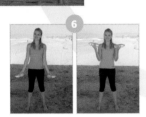

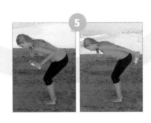

Exercise frequency: 3-4x per week

Speed of movement: 2-1-2 seconds: That means 2 seconds from the starting position to the final position. Hold the final position for 1 second, and then return to the starting position within 2 seconds.

Set duration: 60 seconds per exercise

Workout:
1. Wall sit, pg. 99
2. Squats, pg. 100
3. 45-degree three-point push-ups, pg. 43
4. Cross-legged squat, pg. 101
5. Triceps press, pg. 96
6. Biceps curls, pg. 93
7. Parachutist push-ups, pg. 50
8. Shoulder stretch, pg. 90

WEEK 4:

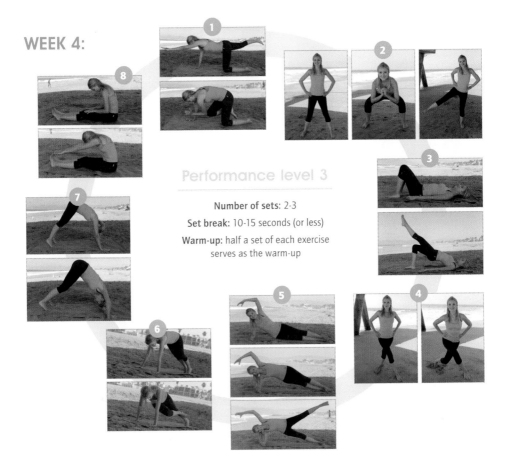

Performance level 3

Number of sets: 2-3
Set break: 10-15 seconds (or less)
Warm-up: half a set of each exercise
serves as the warm-up

Exercise frequency: 4x per week

Speed of movement: 2-1-2 seconds: That means 2 seconds from the starting position to the final position. Hold the final position for 1 second, and then return to the starting position within 2 seconds.

Set duration: 60 seconds per exercise

Workout:
1. Diagonal all-fours position + crunch, pg. 88
2. Squat + side kick, pg. 103
3. Bridge + leg extension, pg. 118
4. Cross-legged squat, pg. 101
5. Extended forearm side plank + leg raise, pg. 71
6. Diagonal mountain climber, pg. 80
7. Parachutist push-ups, pg. 50
8. Seated back stretch, pg. 124

WEEK 5:

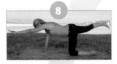
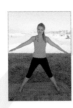
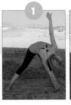

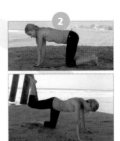
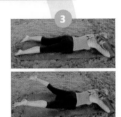

Performance level 3

Number of sets: 2-3

Set break: 10-15 seconds (or less)

Warm-up: half a set of each exercise
serves as the warm-up

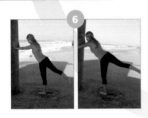

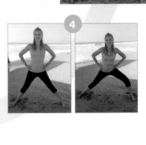
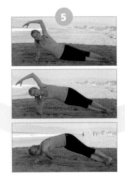

Exercise frequency: 4x per week

Speed of movement: 3-1-3 seconds: That means 3 seconds from the starting position to the final position. Hold the final position for 1 second, and then return to the starting position within 3 seconds.

Set duration: 60 seconds per exercise

Workout:
1. Crossover reach, pg. 123
2. 90-degree back kick, pg. 110
3. Prone position + hip extension, pg. 120
4. Side lunge, pg. 106
5. Extended forearm side plank + twist, pg. 72
6. 45-degree three-point push-ups, pg. 43
7. Lateral raise, pg. 94
8. All-fours position + diagonal extension, pg. 87

159

WEEK 6:

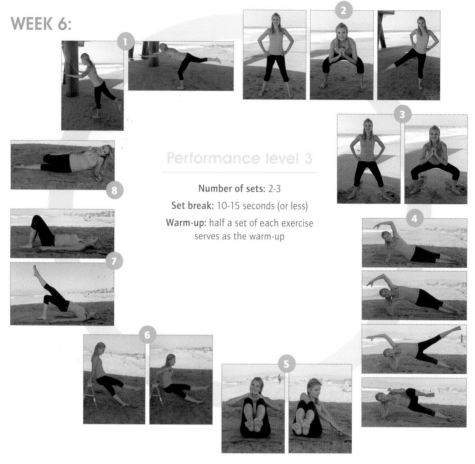

Performance level 3

Number of sets: 2-3

Set break: 10-15 seconds (or less)

Warm-up: half a set of each exercise serves as the warm-up

Exercise frequency: 4x per week

Speed of movement: 3-1-3 seconds: That means 3 seconds from the starting position to the final position. Hold the final position for 1 second, and then return to the starting position within 3 seconds.

Set duration: 60 seconds per exercise

Workout:
1. Standing scale, pg. 117
2. Squat + side kick, pg. 103
3. Plié squats, pg. 104
4. Forearm side plank + crunch, pg. 74
5. Advanced seated crunch, pg. 85
6. Three-point dips, pg. 52
7. Bridge + leg extension, pg. 118
8. Side quadriceps stretch, pg. 129

WEEK 7: *CORE WEEK*

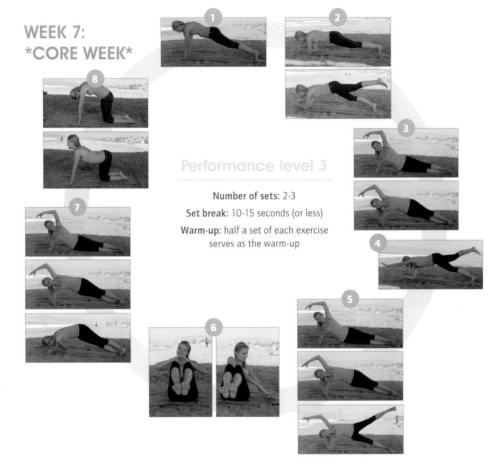

Performance level 3

Number of sets: 2-3
Set break: 10-15 seconds (or less)
Warm-up: half a set of each exercise serves as the warm-up

Exercise frequency: 4x per week

Speed of movement: 3-1-3 seconds: That means 3 seconds from the starting position to the final position. Hold the final position for 1 second, and then return to the starting position within 3 seconds.

Set duration: 60 seconds per exercise

Workout:
1. Full plank, pg. 60
2. Forearm plank + leg extension, pg. 58
3. Extended forearm side plank, pg. 70
4. Forearm plank + diagonal extension pg. 60
5. Extended forearm side plank + leg raise, pg. 71
6. Advanced seated crunch, pg. 85
7. Extended forearm side plank + twist, pg. 72
8. Cat-cow, pg. 97

WEEK 8: *TIGHT BUNS WEEK*

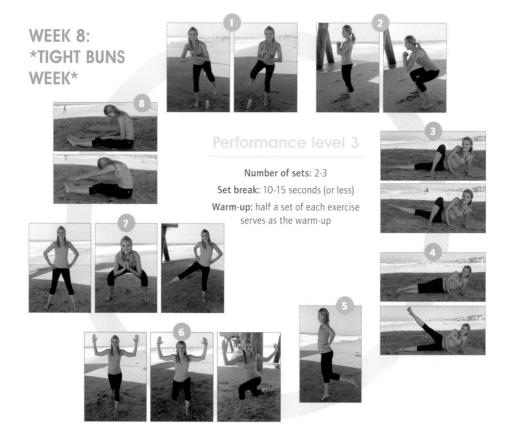

Performance level 3

Number of sets: 2-3
Set break: 10-15 seconds (or less)
Warm-up: half a set of each exercise serves as the warm-up

Exercise frequency: 4x per week

Speed of movement: 3-1-3 seconds: That means 3 seconds from the starting position to the final position. Hold the final position for 1 second, and then return to the starting position within 3 seconds.

Set duration: 60 seconds per exercise

Workout:
1. Left-right leaps, pg. 98
2. Squats, pg. 100
3. Side adduction, pg. 122
4. Side abduction, pg. 121
5. One-legged heel raises, pg. 109
6. Lunge + rotation, pg. 108
7. Squat + side kick, pg. 103
8. Seated back stretch, pg. 124

WEEK 9: FINAL PHASE I

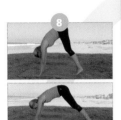
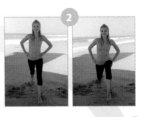
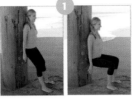
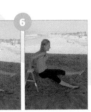
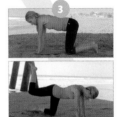
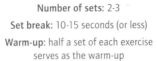
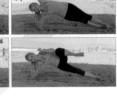
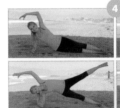
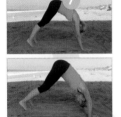
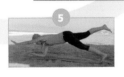

Performance level 3

Number of sets: 2-3
Set break: 10-15 seconds (or less)
Warm-up: half a set of each exercise serves as the warm-up

Exercise frequency: 4x per week

Speed of movement: 4-1-4 seconds: That means 4 seconds from the starting position to the final position. Hold the final position for 1 second, and then return to the starting position within 4 seconds.

Set duration: 65 seconds per exercise

Workout:
1. Wall sit, pg. 99
2. Forward lunge, pg. 107
3. 90-degree back kick, pg. 110
4. Forearm side plank + crunch, pg. 74
5. Forearm plank + diagonal extension, pg. 60
6. Three-point dips, pg. 52
7. Parachutist push-ups, pg. 50
8. Hand-to-foot stretch, pg. 126

WEEK 10: FINAL PHASE II

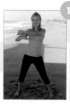
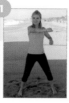
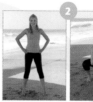
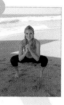

Performance level 3

Number of sets: 2-3
Set break: 10-15 seconds (or less)
Warm-up: half a set of each exercise serves as the warm-up

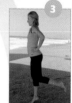

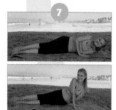

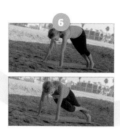

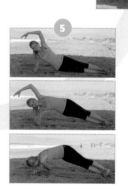

Exercise frequency: 4x per week

Speed of movement: 4-1-4 seconds: That means 4 seconds from the starting position to the final position. Hold the final position for 1 second, and then return to the starting position within 4 seconds.

Set duration: 65 seconds per exercise

Workout:
1. Shadowboxing, pg. 40
2. Toe squats, pg. 102
3. One-legged heel raises, pg. 109
4. Forearm plank + diagonal extension, pg. 60
5. Extended forearm side plank + twist, pg. 72
6. Diagonal mountain climber, pg. 80
7. Arm extension on your side, pg. 53
8. Crossover reach, pg. 123

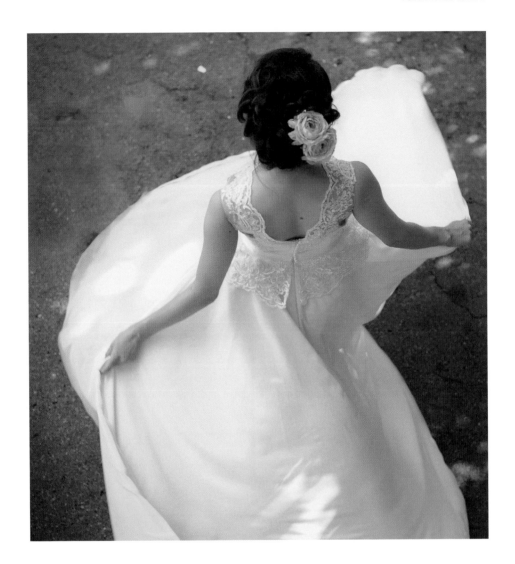

8 NUTRITION

ON LOVE ALONE

8 Nutrition: Because You Can't Live on Love Alone

Dr. Gabriele Anderl began practicing medicine in 1989. Since 1998, Dr. Anderl has been in private practice for nutritional medicine and each year she uses her expert knowledge to guide people to their desired weight. She also serves as the medical representative for nutritional medicine at the German Society for Nutritional Medicine and has successfully led nutrition seminars with several hundred participants. Dr. Anderl is excited to share the secrets of a constructive diet with you for the Perfect Wedding Workout.

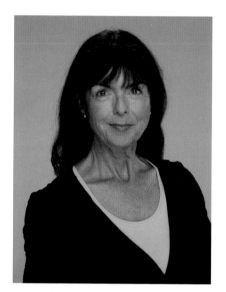

Dr. Gabriele Anderl,
nutritional expert

8.1 DIET MYTHS AND CLARIFICATION

#1 Carbohydrates make you fat.

This assertion is only partly true. Carbohydrates that are quickly absorbed by the body, such as simple sugars (glucose, fructose, sugar, etc.) and white flour products (rolls, pretzels, pizza dough, etc.) quickly raise the insulin level. If the generated energy is not burned, it is stored in the form of fat, and thus results in weight gain. Vegetables and salads are also in the carbohydrate group. These foods generally supply little energy, but instead give us lots of nutrients. Vegetables and salads are perfectly suited for losing excess weight.

#2 Five meals are better than three

It depends on the individual. People who are chronically ill, malnourished, or have had gastro-intestinal surgery, along with tumor patients and immunosuppressed individuals are better able to meet their higher energy needs (and nutritional needs) with five meals and should likely gain weight, or at least not lose weight.

Overweight people, or anyone looking to lose weight, should keep their insulin level on fasting. This is achieved by fasting for several hours between meals. Three meals allow the insulin level to regulate itself, which is the basic requirement for reducing depot fat, or adipose tissue. In-between meals or eating constantly often leads to weight gain.

8.2 THE WEDDING WORKOUT NUTRITIONAL PROGRAM

Who doesn't wish to experience their most important day with vigor and vitality while feeling beautiful and irresistible?

In addition to the workout, nutrition plays an important role here. It is common knowledge that beauty comes from within. Some food ingredients are aphrodisiacs, while others have health-enhancing properties. Many, particularly plant-based foods, keep us fit and lean while others make us fat.

This program allows you to lose weight in a healthy way without feeling hungry, and to feel great and beautiful for the most beautiful day of your life!

We will share two important tips with you here: Be a good sport and keep a sense of humor! No one is born a master. And take your time! Go through the program chapter by chapter and work on the tasks of each respective chapter.

If you start out highly motivated and focused on your goal, create your individual approach, and adhere to a few nutritional principles (What do I eat when? How much, and why?), you will be fitter and leaner in just a few weeks.

8.2.1 Motivation, motivation, motivation

Start your Wedding Workout nutrition program with a serious question: "Why do I want to lose weight?" You might think it strange to consider this question for more than a brief moment so close to your wedding, but an honest answer to this question is critical to your success.

Focus on this question! What really motivates you? What do you associate with the concept of fewer pounds on the scale? How do you see yourself when you are thinner? What feelings do you associate with a new, lower weight?

Imagine what it would feel like to weigh less, for your clothes to fit better, or to wear a smaller size. Think about you as a vision in white!

PRACTICE TIP

- Pack a backpack with a 5 kg weight and one with a 10 kg weight. Wear the 5 kg backpack for at least two hours during your day (for instance, while doing housework); wear the 10 kg backpack to briskly climb two to three flights of stairs. After you take off these backpacks, you will have a good idea of what it might feel like to be 5 or 10 kg lighter.

- Compare current photos with older ones, of when you were thinner. Hanging those photos in a prominent place can be helpful and motivating.

- Find buddies who will mentally support you. Share your plan with your best friend or your colleagues.

TASK:

Find at least THREE good reasons why you personally wish to lose weight—for yourself— and why you are willing to accept the struggles and deprivations. They should be personal reasons that stem from you and that are not solely related to your wedding.

Write these reasons down! Phrase them like this: "I want to lose weight because" or "I want to be leaner and lighter because."

8.2.2 Setting goals

Define YOUR goal in numbers, clearly and explicitly. Set a time frame as well. (It will likely be the timespan up to your wedding.)

For long-term success, it is important to tackle the weight loss now, but it is also important to understand that it needs to be a lifelong task.

You can be ambitious, but remain realistic!

PRACTICE TIP

- When was the last time you were at your target weight? The longer ago it was, the more difficult it will be to reach again.

- You can expect approximately one kg per month of reduced fat weight. Some of you will be disappointed because shady advertising often promises more.

But don't worry: There are some tricks to force more weight loss (see the Low Carb section), but there are NO silver bullets! That is the bad news. And now for the good news: it's up to YOU! If you meticulously follow all recommendations and complete your workout regularly, your efforts will be met with success.

But don't cheat yourself! You have to be honest with yourself, but not too strict (see the Relapse Prevention section).

TASK:
Zero in on your goal and write it down! For instance, I will lose 5 kg within 6 months!

PRACTICE TIP

Reward yourself! Even for accomplished sub-goals. BUT: The rewards cannot be eating or drinking.

For instance: After one month, you will have one kg less on the scale. Treat yourself and your intended to a movie date.

BEWARE OF THE TRAP

Keep your body-building plan, but jettison your unrealistic expectations as quickly as possible! If you are the Rubenesque body type with a curvy bottom, hips, and thighs, you will also lose weight in these areas but your basic silhouette will not change to a lean, athletic type.

But combined with the right workout, you will be able to look forward to a leaner and tighter body shape!

8.2.3 Relapse prevention

No one is born a master! Be a good sport and get ready for a long journey—a new path you will NEVER leave. But long-term your path may include the odd detour, meaning your weight-loss action can stall, or you might even gain back a little weight.

That's when it is important to remember the emergency plan (i.e., relapse prevention).

It's a familiar scenario: You made a commitment and then something gets in the way.

What matters now is not to give up, but to keep going! You pick up where you left off. Every pound you lost matters. Defend your success! Also keep rereading your motivation and your goal, and then draft a relapse letter along with a contract with yourself.

TASK:
Draft an actual contract with everything that belongs in a contract (see chapter 4).

You absolutely MUST sign this contract with yourself! Keep it in a safe place only you have access to, but where you can read it anytime you like.

We are just human and have weak moments. You need such a binding contract to bring you back during those weak moments, when you think that it's all for nothing or it just takes too long, or your fellow humans make it difficult for you to lose weight. Not true!

Prove those haters wrong!

ANYONE CAN LOSE WEIGHT! As long as they have the will—and some important information.

8.2.4 Taking stock: The status quo and the issue of want or must?

First, resolve the question of whether you *want* to lose weight, *have* to lose weight, or *should* lose weight.

The body mass index (BMI) will help you figure out if you are a normal weight or over-weight. For this calculation, you need your actual weight in kg or pounds and your exact height in centimeters or inches. Your body height squared is your approximate body sur-face area. Now divide your weight by your body surface area.

$$BMI = kg / cm2 \text{ or } lbs / in2$$

If your BMI is below 25, you should not lose weight. If it is above 25 but below 30, you could work on losing a little weight (3 to 5 kg). If your BMI is above 30, some weight loss is advisable for health reasons.

At this point, please note that weight-loss recommendations only apply to otherwise he-althy persons. If you are suffering from a chronic illness—particularly diabetes mellitus or heart, liver, or kidney disease—you should not participate in this program.

On principal, written recommendations are not a substitute for a personal consultation with a physician.

8.2.5 Desire and reality: The issue of energy balance

The fact is that a person eating more than he can burn in a day (in the form of calories) will gain weight. If he eats less than he needs to maintain his status quo, he will lose weight. If the energy demand and supply are equal, weight remains constant.

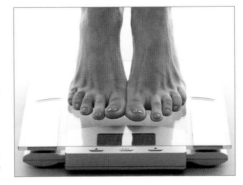

Thus, the question of whether or not you will lose weight is a matter of energy ba-lance.

What you need is a negative energy balan-ce. How do you create a negative energy balance? The unfortunate truth is that you have to eat less than you need.

Since a person's exact energy expenditure cannot be ascertained without the use of elaborate measuring devices and you most likely don't know yours, we must resort to general recommendations. Research has taught us that to lose weight we must cut out at least 350 calories per day.

This program only gives you ten weeks. Try to cut out 500 calories each day, especially if your goals are ambitious. If you read chapters 6 and 7, you already know how to go about this.

But—and this is really important—DON'T COUNT calories! Counting calories only leads to frustration and not the desired weight. Get a feel for your body and your energy requirements and keep reading!

If I periodically refer to kcal, it is because in the end weight loss is the result of a decreased supply of energy-rich foods that contain carbohydrates, protein, and fat.

Approximately 7,000 kcal are stored in one kg of fat tissue. So if you cut out 500 kcal each day, you can cut out 3,500 kcal a week (7 x 500 kcal) and lose about one half kg of depot fat.

To make sure you really lose fat and not muscle, you should definitely not stop eating, meaning do not embark on a starvation diet. Make sure you take in an adequate supply of protein-rich foods during each phase (also see 8.2.7)!

If you diligently follow all of the recommendations and rev up your metabolism, you can lose up to 2 kg of depot fat in 4 weeks. (There are, however, people who lose fat more slowly or more quickly. The determining variables here are genetics, muscle mass, age, etc.)

If you continue the calculation, you will end up with a possible weight loss—or rather depot fat loss—of 5 kg in 10 weeks. But please try not to overdo it or get upset if in your case it is less than that!

Sometimes weight loss can be slow to start, but still works over an extended period of time. That is also why you should stick with it after the wedding, especially if your starting BMI is above 30. It will be worth it!

8.2.6 Cutting out unnecessary energy: First steps

Now that you have read this far, I hope you cannot wait to get started. You can and you should!

As a first step, banish all foods that ONLY offer energy but contain few nutrients, especially micronutrients (also see 8.2.7).

It is about the energy-nutrient balance of each INDIVIDUAL food, or rather about the energy density to nutrient density ratio. Amino acids, trace elements, vitamins, minerals, and phytochemicals are so-called *essential nutrients* our body cannot produce on its own and we must therefore eat every day.

The higher the nutrient share, the better!

In other words, foods that contain too much fat or sugar provide primarily energy, meaning they are NOT SUITABLE for weight loss. I like to call these foods empty calories or energy cardboard.

On principal, there are NO forbidden foods. Nevertheless, you should avoid the following products for at least the first four weeks of the power phase!

Energy-dense foods:

- Beverages that contain sugar (all regular soft drinks, juices, sports drinks, and other so-called reduced-calorie light beverages, etc.)

- Alcoholic beverages (beer, wine, hard liquor, liqueurs, cocktails, champagne, reduced-alcohol beverages, non-alcoholic beer)

- Cake, pastries, cookies, pretzels

- Chocolate, gummy bears, ice cream (milk and water-based)

- Fatty meat and sausage products (pork belly, spare ribs, pork butt, meatloaf, veal sausage, mortadella, salami, liverwurst, most cold cuts)

- High-fat dairy products (cheese with more than 30% fat content, cream, crème fraiche, mascarpone, milk with more than 3.8% fat content, full-fat yogurt)

- "Dairy" products like fruit yogurt, fruit buttermilk, etc.; pizza, burgers, French fries, etc.

You should NOT eat any of these foods for at least the first four weeks!

8.2.7 The essentials about nutrients

Food is essential. Our food contains more than 50 *essential nutrients*. These include some protein building blocks like amino acids, vitamins (e.g., vitamins A, B, C, D, E, and K), minerals (e.g., magnesium, calcium), and trace elements (e.g., selenium, zinc). Our body cannot produce any of these essential micronutrients, so it must rely on a regular—ideally daily—supply. A lack of or inadequate supply of these micronutrients results in a state of severe deficiency that can affect our metabolic processes and can even lead to illness.

Micronutrients are to our body what spark plugs are to an engine. Even a car with a full gas tank won't start without spark plugs.

Macronutrients—carbohydrates, protein, and fat—supply the energy our cells need to start metabolic processes. To stay with the image of a car engine, macronutrients are like different types of fuel: regular, super, and diesel.

Macronutrients supply energy, meaning they have calories, while micronutrients do not themselves supply energy but are essential catalysts for energy extraction (i.e., the burning of calories). It would be wrong to cut them out because that would impede all metabolic processes like, for instance, fat burning.

An ideal meal should be based on the principles of the LOGI pyramid (you can find it online).

> **Rule of thumb:** 50 to 70 g of carbohydrates + 20 to 25 g of protein + 15 to 20 g of fat per meal

Foods that are high in carbohydrates are listed later in this section.

Foods that are high in protein are meat, fish, legumes (lentils, beans, peas), eggs, dairy products (milk, yogurt, cheese), and whole grains.

Please note that many high-protein foods contain hidden fats, particularly cheese and sausage. Since sausage tends to be relatively high in fat and salt, it is not conducive to weight loss. I recommend completely eliminating sausage and sausage products for at least these ten weeks. (In paragraph 8.2.6, we already temporarily eliminated prepared foods, pizza, cake, cookies, and snacks—all of which tend to be high in fat—from your menu).

Plant-based foods tend to have a higher nutrient content as well as lower energy content. They also supply important protectants like phytochemicals (e.g., carotenoids, flavonoids, anthocyanins, and many more).

The ideal diet places emphasis on plant-based foods and includes meat twice a week, fish twice a week, and vegetarian meals three times a week.

The typical Mediterranean or Asian cuisine offers many suggestions. To find lots of good recipes, do an online search with the keywords "eat smarter."

> **Rule of thumb for protein intake:** 20 g of protein per meal in the form of 100 g of meat or fish, or low-fat quark (curd).

> **Rule of thumb for fat intake:** 15 to 20 g total per meal in the form of 3 teaspoons of oil, 3 tablespoons of cream, 20 g of butter, or 2 eggs.

> **PRACTICE TIP:**
>
> Whenever possible, eat foods with high nutrient density (and low energy density)!
>
> Plant-based foods are particularly beneficial, especially vegetables, fruit, seeds, nuts, and appropriate amounts of whole-grain products, particularly oats, oat bran, and millet (flakes), as well as amaranth and quinoa.

Modern science has determined that we would need to consume 2 kg of fresh vegetables and fruit each day to cover our protectants requirement (e.g., antioxidants, etc.).

> **PRACTICE TIP:**
>
> Eat at least five servings of organic vegetables and fruit each day, preferably in the traffic-light colors (red, yellow, and green). Give preference to local and regional produce and eat colorful!

To cut down on fat, brush the skillet with 1 teaspoon of oil (never pour oil directly from the bottle onto food or into the skillet), use spray bottles for salad dressing, buy reduced-fat versions of dairy products and cheese, replace butter with quark (curd), replace cream with sour cream, and roast and cook food at low temperatures. Stewing and steaming requires little fat and protects vitamins!

Which type of fat should you use? Today's gold standard is rapeseed oil, which is available as high-quality oil (non-GMO, cold-pressed) with or without butter flavor at the supermarket. The latter can even be brushed or drizzled onto wholegrain bread to replace butter.

Rapeseed oil has a burn point of 200° C/392° F, so it can be used for frying. Its fatty acid structure is an ideal blend of a monounsaturated fatty acid and polyunsaturated fatty acids (omega-3 and omega-6), but it does not change the rule of thumb of 3 teaspoons per meal.

Omega-3 fatty acids are scarce in our diet, but they are particularly beneficial to our health and beauty, and should therefore be held in high regard.

Other good sources of omega-3 fatty acids are flaxseed oil and walnut oil (only use cold!) and fatty fish like tuna, herring, mackerel, and salmon.

Indulge yourself at least once a week with a portion of fatty fish!

CARBOHYDRATES				
Food	Carbohydrates in g			
	40	50	60	70
Wholegrain rolls	90 g	115 g	135 g	160 g
Wholegrain bread	110 g	135 g	160 g	190 g
Wheat rolls	80 g	100 g	115 g	135 g
Oats	70 g	90 g	105 g	125 g
Wholegrain pasta, raw	70 g	85 g	100 g	115 g
Brown rice, raw	55 g	70 g	80 g	95 g
Boiled potatoes, with skin	270 g	335 g	400 g	470 g

The table tells you how many grams of carbohydrates a food supplies (e.g., a slice of wholegrain bread that weighs 110 g provides 40g of carbohydrates).

Particularly during the power phase (weeks 1 to 4), it is important to only consume carbohydrates in the morning, and consume them sparingly.

Of course, your body size and hunger—or rather satiation—are also major factors.

If you are 160 cm (5' 2") or smaller, 40-50 g of carbohydrates at breakfast should be sufficient. If you are 170 cm (5' 6") or taller, you can consume 60-70 g. NEVER eat high-carb foods in-between meals because this will interfere with fat burning.

During the transition phase (weeks 9 and 10), you can proceed according to your wishes or the weight you have reached at that point.

If you are planning on losing more weight, you should extend the transition phase. If you have already reached your personal goal, you can now begin to also eat high-carb foods in the evening, but proceed with caution and initially don't exceed 40 g of carbs so you don't jeopardize your success.

The goal for the holding phase (weeks 10+) is for you to stabilize your weight, meaning the weight you can maintain long-term, with a balanced mixed diet that contains, on average, 60 g of carbs per meal. (Factors such as body size, age, muscle mass, basal metabolic rate, activity level, etc., of course continue to also play a role.)

FAT		
Per portion	Food	Fat content (in g)
Milk and dairy products		
1 glass (0.2 l)	Whole milk (3.5%)	7
1 glass (0.2 l)	Low-fat milk (1.5%)	3
100 g	Quark (curd) (40%)	11
100 g	Quark (curd) (10%)	2
1 Tbsp.	Whipping cream 30%	8
1 Tbsp.	Sour cream 10%	2
1 slice (30 g)	Gouda 45%	5
1 slice (30 g)	Gouda 30%	2
Meat and sausage		
125 g	Pork butt	17
125 g	Pork tenderloin	3
125 g	Duck	21
125 g	Turkey	1
30 g	Salami	9
30 g	Cooked ham	1

Bread and baked goods		
1	Croissant	25
1 slice	Wholegrain bread	1
Sides (e.g., potatoes)		
1 serving 200 g	Fried potatoes	16
1 serving 200 g	Boiled potatoes	0
Total		119

All items shaded in green are a good, low-fat alternative with the same portion size.

That means if you make smart choices, you don't have to give up anything, but over the course of the day, you cut out a ton of energy and jumpstart fat burning.

All of the foods listed above can be eaten in one day. If you choose the reduced-fat version—the green version—you have cut out 104 g of fat in one day. That is the equivalent of more than 900 kcal or approximately two meals.

A sample daily plan

This is what your day might look like:

Morning

	Protein	Carbs
1 glass buttermilk (0.2 l)	7 g	8 g
150 g yogurt, 1.5%	5 g	7 g
125 g quark (curd), 20%	10 g	7 g
1 egg	8 g	-
50 g rolled oats	5 g	30 g
Subtotal	35 g	52 g

Lunch

	Protein	Carbs
125 g veal tenderloin/ 150 g Halibut	25 g/30 g	-
200 g broccoli	7 g	5 g
100 g butter lettuce	2 g	2 g
Subtotal	34 g/39 g	7 g

Dinner

	Protein	Carbs
200 turkey breast fillet	40 g	-
100 g butter lettuce	2 g	2 g
Subtotal	42 g	2 g
Total	111 g/116 g	61 g

You can vary this sample plan at your discretion. Use different types of meat and eat lots of different vegetables. (All vegetables are beneficial. With salads and vegetables, you DON'T have to worry about the quantity if you only use 2-3 teaspoons of oil during preparation.)

On vegetarian days, use legumes, tofu, quark, nuts, seeds, and whole grains, as well as amaranth and quinoa as protein sources.

If you forgo classic sides—bread, rice, pasta, potatoes—for lunch and dinner during the power phase (first 4 weeks), you will really rev up fat burning.

For lunches during the transition phase—weeks 5 to 8—you can allow yourself either a small side (also see carbohydrate table, e.g., 20-30 carbs) or a corresponding amount of fruit for dessert (e.g., 150 g pineapple, 2 medium apples, 1 banana, 200 g blueberries, 200 g cherries, or 4-5 tangerines contain 20-30 carbs).

8.2.8 Your personal formula

Every person is a unique individual and each person's excess weight has different reasons and causes. You should be aware of some of the main catalysts so you can purposefully counteract them.

Have you already eaten today? Why? Were you hungry? Did you have a craving? Or were you bored, sad, or frustrated, or was it just out of habit? There are many reasons.

In nutritional psychology, we refer to regulatory levels of eating behavior. The most important ones are:

- Hunger/craving

- Satiation

- Meal rhythm

- Choice and amount of consumed foods

- Joy, sadness, frustration, stress

- Habits

- Exercise/sports

- Social environment, cultural imprint, vacation, communal eating, meal invitations, etc.

Every day, each of these factors influences what we eat, why we eat, and how much we eat.

To successfully lose weight, the meal rhythm is the most important.

Eat three times a day! DO NOT eat between meals! Do not have chewing gum, crackers, gummy bears, or even healthy things like fruit.

> **PRACTICE TIP:**
>
> Eat three meals a day, breakfast, lunch, and dinner. DO NOT eat between meals.
>
> Only drink water, preferably still mineral water (with plenty of hydrogen carbonate, magnesium, and calcium). That little hunger in-between meals is usually just thirst!

Drinking water promotes fat burning! Water is a true fat burner and our most important food since our bodies are more than 70% water.

8.2.9 Let's go!: The power phase (weeks 1-4)

Your first four weeks are the power phase. Before you get started, please review all PRACTICE TIPS from sections 1 through 8.

You are highly motivated, focused on your goal; have stocked up on lots of mineral water, vegetables, fruit, and lettuce; have hidden the crackers, chips, and beer in the basement or given them to the neighbors, and are now ready to eat just three times a day.

Now let's get started!

The first four weeks are low-carb weeks. That means you will consume relatively few carbs.

What are carbohydrates and in which foods can they be found?
Carbohydrates is a collective term for all types of sugar and sugar compounds such as glucose, fructose, lactose, sugar, and starch, the so-called *polysaccharides*.

Carbohydrates can be found in sugar, soft drinks, juices, fruit, rice, pasta, potatoes, rolled oats, etc.

Try to avoid sugar as much as possible, and use artificial sweetener or Stevia if you want to sweeten your tea or coffee.

During these first four weeks, you should also avoid the classic sides like rice, pasta, and potatoes. Eat carbohydrates for breakfast to supply your brain and nervous system with the necessary fuel.

Eat bread sparingly! Try to make friends with some rolled oat muesli for breakfast. Rolled oats contain very little sugar, but do have 14 g of protein, 11 g of fiber, and many beneficial micronutrients (vitamin B1, magnesium, iron, zinc, etc.) per 100 g of oats. Fiber is important for intestinal flora and intestinal motility.

Keep your eyes open at the grocery store! Lots of prepared muesli contains sugar, too many raisins (sugar), too much fat (coconut flakes, chocolate flakes), or other less beneficial ingredients. Just buy oats (steel cut or rolled, depending on your preference) and mix your own muesli with spelt flakes, millet flakes (open package must be refrigerated), flax seed, walnuts, hazelnuts (ten nuts), sesame (1-2 tsp.), pumpkin seeds, chia seeds, dried fruit (e.g., 1-2 unsulfured dried apricots), or fresh fruit.

> **Rule of thumb:** 5 generous tablespoons of rolled oats equal about 50 g with 25-30 carbohydrates. Add 20 g oat bran (3 generous tablespoons supply 8 g carbohydrates) and one piece of fruit (a diced apple, pear, or nectarine, or a handful of berries provides approximately 15 g carbohydrates)..

You can soak the muesli the night before (if you use steel-cut oats) or pour some 1.5% milk over it shortly before breakfast. Unsweetened oat drink (a slightly sweet taste) or rice milk are also good choices. Oat drink contains 6 g of carbs per 100 ml, while rice milk contains 4.9 g of carbs per 100 ml.

If we now add up the listed amount of carbs, we get a total of 60 g.

That is ideal for one meal. You should continue this breakfast during the other phases as well. You can vary the liquids, the individual grain components, fruits, seeds, and nuts. Depending on the time of year, you can also use different spices and herbs, like fresh mint in summer or cinnamon and cardamom in winter.

Your muesli will have 13 g of protein when made with oat drink, and 16 g when made with milk.

The amount of protein that will allow you to feel satiated and maintain muscle is 20-25 g per meal.

One hundred grams of low-fat quark (curd) provides 13 g of protein. You can just eat it plain (low-fat quark crème has a nice consistency). If you find regular quark too dense, stir in some mineral water. You can also add flavor ingredients, but do not add any sugar. You can also stir the quark into the muesli.

> **PRACTICE TIP:**
>
> Avoid fruit teas as the dried fruit releases sugar.
>
> Large amounts of coffee can intensify hunger feelings and cause an excess of gastric acid. It is better to drink tea! Black and especially green tea contain substances that promote fat burning!

Enjoy your meals! Eat slowly and engage all of your senses!

Enjoy the sight of an appetizing meal arranged on a plate, inhale the aroma that reaches your nostrils, taste the food, chew slowly (ten times for each bite) and with relish, and only then swallow it!

You can find all the ingredients at any full-service supermarket or at an organic food store. If possible, buy organic products, especially fruits and vegetables.

Use lots of fresh herbs to provide additional vitamins and minerals. Lemon (juice, grated lemon peel, or zest) and ginger (chopped) intensify the flavor and improve digestion.

One serving of Bircher muesli requires:

- 5 tablespoons steel cut oats (soak overnight in double the amount of water and chill)
- Juice from ½ organic lemon
- 1 tablespoon heavy cream
- 1 apple, unpeeled (grate coarsely and mix in)
- 5 chopped nuts (hazelnuts, walnuts, or almonds) for garnish

What about the bread lovers? They should buy wholegrain bread and avoid white flour products.

One slice of wholegrain bread (45 g) provides approximately 20 g of carbs, so you can eat three slices of bread (providing you don't use jam or honey), or you can eat two slices and still have room for 2 teaspoons of jam and a piece of fruit.

Take a look at the **carbohydrate table** to learn more.

With respect to the make-up of your meals, you can use the sample daily plan as a guide. It contains few carbs, but a higher than average amount of protein. You won't reach that every day—particularly not on meatless days, when protein intake tends to be less.

The sample plan shows you what you can eat to lose weight and maintain muscle successfully without going hungry.

8.2.10 Transition phase (weeks 5-8)

Eat the same breakfasts as during the power phase. Eat your lunch 4-6 hours after breakfast to optimize fat burning. Make sure your lunch consists of 100-150 g of a protein supplier (fish or meat) and plenty of vegetables. Use only 2-3 teaspoons of rapeseed oil as a cooking and frying fat (or olive oil or walnut oil as an alternative for cold food). Supplement your meal with a small amount of carbs (40 to 50 g maximum) in the form of a side (see carbohydrate table), a fruit dessert, or a smoothie (rule of thumb: a serving of fruit is something that fits into one hand or two handfuls of berries).

8.2.11 Target phase (weeks 9-10)

Your personal wishes or goal and the weight you have reached at this point determine your next steps.

Have you reached your goal? Then enjoy a small amount of carbs, even in the evening. Begin with 40 to 50 g maximum. Choose whole grains, legumes, or potatoes. Fruit is not recommended in the evening because it is relatively high in sugar and will negatively impact metabolism (insulin release).

Have you not reached your goal yet? Have you set new goals, or are you simply enjoying your weight loss so much that you wish to continue? Then continue the transition phase.

Whether or not you have met your goal, three days before the wedding you should switch to the target phase and increase your carbohydrate intake to three times a day. The big day will be strenuous and you will most likely have a drink or two, so it is advisable to get the body used to more carbs again.

8.2.12 Holding phase (weeks 10+)

You have learned a lot and worked hard, and you have succeeded!

Congratulations!

However, it is important not to fall back into bad habits. It is impossible to change in only 10 weeks the behaviors we have practiced and learned over many years, so stick with it! You can switch back to the transition phase any time, or into the target phase to maintain your weight.

You should not stay in the power phase for a long period of time or repeat it in short successions, because the body will adjust to the reduced carbohydrate supply and the effect fizzles.

The three-meals principle continues during the holding phase, but now you should also think about the other regulating factors of eating behavior (see section 8.2.8) and work on one level after another. To do so, I recommend appropriate nutrition coaching like the kind that has been taught successfully in my classes for the past 15 years.

For those of you who are now interested in learning more on this subject matter, I recommend a food nutrition chart to start. There you can look up the nutritional value of all common foods separated by protein, carbohydrates, and fat content per serving—or by weight, fiber content, and amount of energy—for all food groups.

The following chapter includes a list of low-carb recipe ideas divided by season. You can add the side dish of your choice as needed.

Finally, I wish with all my heart that the undertaking you chose in preparation for the most beautiful day of your life will become a permanent success!

Regards,

Dr. Gabriele Anderl

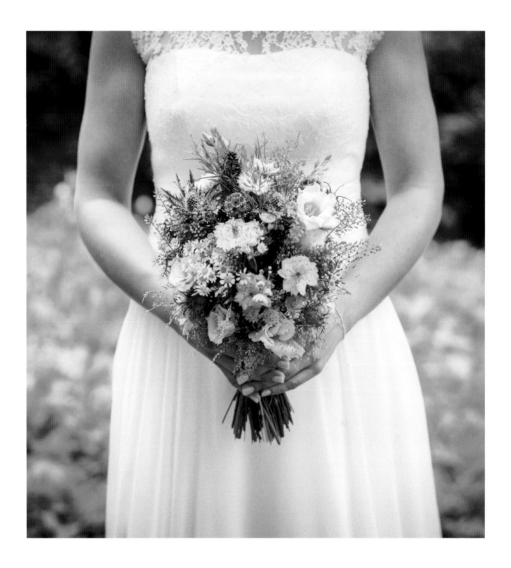

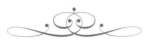

9 MICHAEL'S
FAVORITE RECIPES

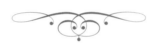

9 Michael's Favorite Recipes

Dr. Gabriele Anderl talked about the essential elements of a constructive diet. People often ask me what I like to eat.

Below are my top 3 favorite recipes for each season.

The quantities listed in the recipes are for one serving. If you plan to cook for your soon-to-be husband, simply double the amounts.

1

ASIAN MANGO AND RED CABBAGE SALAD

Ingredients:

- 175 g (6 oz.) red cabbage
- ½ tsp. honey
- 125 g (4 oz.) onions
- ¼ Tbsp. lemon juice
- ½ Tbsp. peanut butter
- 1Tbsp. oil
- 100 g (4 oz.) mango
- Cilantro
- ¼ Tbsp. roasted sesame seeds
- Salt and pepper

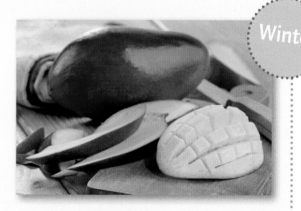

Winter

Preparation:

1. Wash the red cabbage and cut it into quarters. Remove the stalk and cut the cabbage into thin ribbons. In a bowl, toss the cabbage with a pinch of salt, honey, and a little pepper for one minute.

2. Finely slice the onion and add to the cabbage. In a second bowl, mix the lemon juice, peanut butter, and oil. Pour over the cabbage and toss well.

3. Peel the mango and cut into thin ribbons and add to the cabbage. Coarsely chop some cilantro and mix it in with the cabbage.

4. Allow the salad to sit for ten minutes before tasting and adding salt if necessary. Sprinkle with roasted sesame seeds.

Pairs well with grilled shrimp or turkey strips.

②
DUCK BREAST ON GLASS NOODLES

Ingredients:

- 37.5 g (1.3 oz.) glass noodles
- ½ duck breast fillet (approximately 250 g / 9 oz.)
- Salt
- Pepper
- ½ miniature salad cucumber
- ½ red onion
- ½ lime
- ½ Tbsp. Thai fish sauce
- ½ Tbsp. soy sauce
- ½ Tsp. honey
- ½ Tsp. sesame oil
- 2 sprigs of Thai basil or mint
- ½ Tbsp. of peanuts

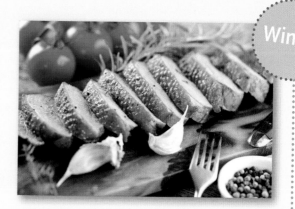

Winter

Preparation:

1. Prepare glass noodles according to package directions. Rinse the duck breast in cold water, pat dry, and make shallow diamond-shaped cuts in the skin with a sharp knife.

2. Place the duck breast in a skillet skin-side down and cook at medium heat until crispy, about 9 minutes. Turn the duck breast over meat-side down. Add pepper and salt to taste and cook for 3 more minutes. Remove the duck from the skillet, wrap it in aluminum foil, and let it rest.

3. Let glass noodles drip dry and use kitchen shears to cut into smaller pieces to your liking. Wash and dry the cucumber, and cut into thin slices. Peel the onion and cut into thin ribbons. Add both ingredients to the noodles.

4. Juice the lime. Mix the lime juice, fish sauce, and honey until well-blended, then whisk in the oil.

5. Mix the sauce and salad ingredients. Thoroughly wash the basil, remove leaves from stems, and finely chop them. Slice the duck breast and plate with the salad. Chop the peanuts and sprinkle on top.

③ POWER BOWL WITH CHICKPEAS - VEGETARIAN

Ingredients:

- 70 g (2.5 oz.) uncooked couscous
- 50 ml (2 oz.) vegetable broth
- 1 small carrot
- 65 g (2.3 oz.) broccoli
- 50 g (2 oz.) radicchio
- ¼ salad cucumber
- 75 g (3 oz.) endive
- 70 g (2.5 oz.) chickpeas
- 1 Tbsp. mixed seeds
- 1 Tbsp. dried cranberries
- 1 Tbsp. cress
- 1 Tbsp. olive oil
- Salt and pepper to taste
- 2 Tbsp. vinaigrette

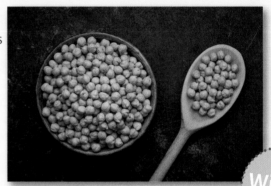

Winte

Preparation:

1. Pour hot water over couscous and let stand for 10 minutes.

2. Wash all other ingredients. Cut the carrot into small pieces, separate the broccoli into small florets, cut the cucumber into thin slices, and cut the radicchio into thin ribbons.

3. Let the chickpeas drain.

4. Heat a little olive oil in a skillet. Sear the carrot pieces and broccoli.

5. Put all ingredients in a bowl and arrange. Recommended: add the salad and couscous first, then the remaining ingredients. Next add the cress, cranberries, and dressing, and season with salt and pepper to taste.

PORK TENDERLOIN WITH ASPARAGUS

Ingredients:

- 100 g (4 oz.) asparagus
- ¼ tsp. salt
- 20 g (3/4 oz.) butter
- ½ egg yolk
- ¼ Tbsp. sherry
- Basil to taste
- ¼ Tbsp. tomato paste
- Lemon juice
- 1 slice pork tenderloin (approximately 150 g / 5 oz.)
- ¾ Tbsp. oil
- Pepper
- Salt
- 1 cherry tomato

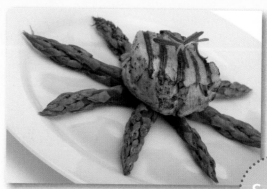

Spring

Preparation:

1. Peel lower third of asparagus stalks (white asparagus must be peeled all the way), trim ends, and cook in boiling salt water until al dente. Drain and keep warm.

2. Melt butter in a saucepan and let it cool slightly. Whisk egg yolk and wine in a double boiler until fluffy. Gradually add the melted butter to the egg yolk mixture.

3. Sear the pork tenderloin in hot oil.

4. Arrange the sauce and asparagus with the pork tenderloin and garnish with the roasted cherry tomato and the basil.

FILLET OF PLAICE WITH SPINACH IN SPICY SAUCE

Ingredients:

- 250 g (9 oz.) fresh spinach
- 1 small red onion
- ½ clove of garlic
- 150 g (5 oz.) fillet of plaice
- 1 Tbsp. oil
- Salt to taste
- Pepper to taste
- Harissa paste to taste

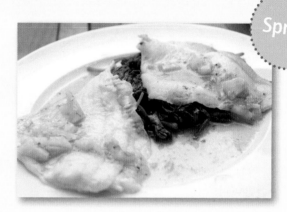

Spring

Preparation:

1. Wash the spinach. Remove stems and tear leaves into smaller pieces. Finely chop onion and garlic, then sauté in oil.

2. Season with salt and pepper, then add the spinach and stir.

3. Season the fillet on both sides with harissa and place it on the spinach.

4. Reduce heat and allow the fish to simmer in the covered skillet.

③ FRITTATA WITH CHARD AND SPELT NOODLES - VEGETARIAN

Spring

Ingredients:

- 25-30 g (1 oz.) whole-grain spelt noodles
- 150 g (5 oz.) chard
- 1 Tbsp. olive oil
- 25 g (1 oz.) pecorino cheese
- 1 egg
- Sea salt
- Pepper

Preparation:

1. Cook spelt noodles and let them cool. Wash the chard and let drain. Remove stems from chard. Cut stems and leaves into wide ribbons.

2. Heat olive oil in a large skillet. Add stems and cook for approximately 5 minutes. Add leaves and cook another 3-5 minutes. Meanwhile grate the pecorino cheese. Mix half of the cheese with the egg and season with salt and pepper to taste.

3. Mix noodles with the chard.

4. Pour egg mixture over noodles and chard and sprinkle with the remaining cheese.

5. Put a lid on the skillet and allow the frittata to set for approximately 15 minutes. The frittata is done when the egg is firm. Finally, sprinkle with more salt and pepper.

Personal recommendation: For a golden-brown and crispy frittata, put it in the oven for 8-10 minutes at 190°C (375° F).

①
MEDITERRANEAN CHICKEN BREAST WITH VEGETABLES

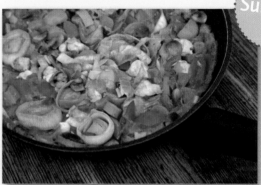

Summe

Ingredients:

- 150 g (5 oz.) chicken breast fillet
- ½ Tbsp. olive oil
- 1 tsp. paprika
- 65 ml (2 oz.) vegetable broth
- ¼ medium onion
- ½ garlic clove
- ½ red pepper (or 1 red and 1 yellow)
- 38 g (1.3 oz.) zucchini
- 25 g (1 oz.) carrots
- 50 g (2 oz.) mushrooms
- 50 g (2 oz.) sour cream
- ¼ glass dry red wine (eliminate for children)
- Fresh basil

- 1½ sprigs of thyme
- Italian-style herbs to taste
- Dried chilies to taste
- Salt and pepper to taste
- Rosemary (fresh or dried) to taste

Preparation:

1. Cut chicken into cubes. Wash vegetables and cube or cut into bite-size pieces. Finely chop garlic and onion. Cut zucchini into thin slices.

2. Heat olive oil in a wok and sear chicken with a little rosemary and paprika powder until crispy. Remove chicken and set aside.

3. Add fresh oil to the wok (or pot) and add vegetables. Sauté for approximately 10 minutes, then deglaze with 65 ml (2 oz.) of vegetable broth. Stir in sour cream and a little red wine. Season to taste with Italian herbs, paprika powder, dried chilies, pepper, and very little salt.

4. Add the chicken and a little basil. Place thyme sprigs on top and simmer in covered wok (pot) for approximately 20 min. Done!

② SALMON WITH SPINACH SALAD AND MANGO

Ingredients:

- 65 g (2 oz.) fresh baby spinach
- ¼ mango
- ½ salmon fillet
- Oil
- ¼ lemon
- 1 small garlic clove
- 10 g (2 Tbsp.) butter
- ¼ red onion

Dressing:

- 1 Tbsp. sweet chili sauce
- ½ Tbsp. soy sauce
- ½ Tbsp. fish sauce
- ½ Tbsp. rice vinegar
- Grated ginger
- 1 Tbsp. sesame oil (light)

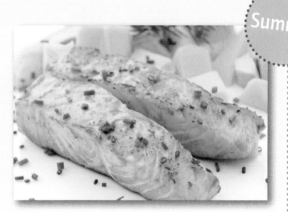

Summer

Preparation:

1. Put a little oil in a skillet and heat (medium heat). Add salmon (skin-side up) and cook until the bottom edges are slightly browned. Carefully flip the salmon. Add butter, garlic, and lemon to the skillet. Allow the butter to briefly foam and the flavors (lemon, garlic) to take effect. Ladle the flavoring ingredients over the salmon with a spoon.

2. Wash and dry the spinach. Remove the mango pit, peel, and cube the fruit. Divide the salmon into bite-size pieces. Peel the onion and cut into thin slices. Arrange everything on two plates.

3. Dressing: Blend the sweet chili sauce, a little ginger, soy sauce, and rice vinegar, then whisk in the oil and season to taste. Drizzle the dressing over the salad and serve.

③ OMELET BURGER WITH ZUCCHINI

Ingredients:

- ½ small zucchini (60 g / 2 oz.)
- 1 sprig Italian parsley
- 1 slice smoked turkey breast (20 g / ¾ oz.)
- 1 egg
- 1 Tbsp. milk (1.5% fat)
- Salt
- Pepper
- 1 Tbsp. rapeseed oil
- 1 whole-grain roll
- 1 Tbsp. quark (curd) with herbs
- 1 lettuce leaf
- 1 small tomato (40 g / 1.5 oz.)

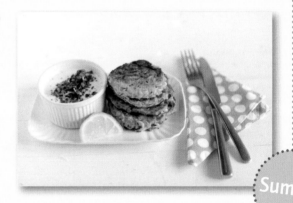

Summe

Preparation:

1. Coarsely grate the zucchini. Wash parsley and shake dry, then pull leaves off the stem and finely chop. Cut the turkey breast into narrow strips. Use a fork to blend egg, milk, a little salt, and pepper in a bowl. Add grated zucchini, parsley, and turkey strips.

2. Heat rapeseed oil in a small skillet and pour in egg mixture. Allow egg mixture to set at low heat for approximately 3 minutes. Flip the omelet and allow the other side to set.

3. Meanwhile, slice the wholegrain roll in half and spread with the quark (curd). Wash the lettuce leaf, shake off water, and place on the bottom half of the roll. Top with the omelet and tuck the edges under or fold the omelet in half.

4. Cut the tomato into thin slices and place on top of the omelet. Top with the remaining half of the roll and enjoy the omelet burger.

BEEF-CASHEW SKILLET

Fall

Ingredients:

- 120 g (4 oz.) beef
- 1 Tbsp. olive oil
- 25-30 g (1 oz.) rice
- ½ bell pepper
- 1 leek
- 1 ½ Tbsp. soy sauce
- 20 g (3/4 oz.) cashews
- Pinch of brown sugar

Preparation:

1. Cut beef into thin diagonal strips and sear in olive oil.

2. Cook rice in salt water.

3. Cut bell pepper and leek into thin ribbons or rings and toss with other ingredients in a bowl.

4. Add all ingredients to the beef in the skillet and sauté. Stir every 3 minutes. Serve with rice.

② RED RADISH AND CRAB SALAD

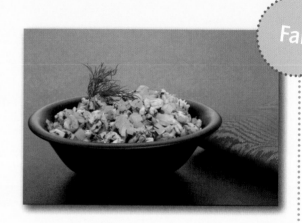

Fall

Ingredients:

- 3 red radishes
- ½ bell pepper
- ¼ onion
- ½ sprig dill
- 35 g (1 oz.) crabmeat
- 1 ½ Tbsp. lemon juice
- ½ Tbsp. olive oil
- Sea salt
- Pepper

Preparation:

1. Wash radishes and slice thinly. Wash bell pepper and cut into small strips.

2. Skin and dice the onion, chop the dill.

3. Place ingredients in a bowl together with the crabmeat and mix with lemon juice and olive oil. Add salt and pepper to taste.

3
ASIAN BROCCOLI SKILLET WITH HONEY TOFU - VEGETARIAN

Ingredients:

- 100 g (3.5 oz.) tofu
- 1 tsp. honey
- 3 tsp. soy sauce
- ½ bell pepper (medium)
- 75 g (3 oz.) broccoli
- ½ leek
- 1 Tbsp. rapeseed oil
- ½ garlic clove
- 1 dash of lime juice
- Salt
- Pepper

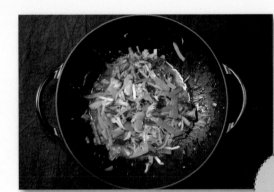

Fall

Preparation:

1. Cut tofu into cubes. Blend honey and soy sauce, add tofu, and let marinate for one hour.

2. Blanch broccoli in salt water, dice the bell pepper, and cut the leek into thin slices. Drain tofu and set marinade aside in a bowl.

3. Put oil in a wok and cook tofu until crispy. Remove tofu from wok and keep warm.

4. Place vegetables in the wok and cook approximately 5 minutes until al dente, then add garlic.

5. Add the remaining marinade and the tofu, season with salt and pepper to taste, and add the lime juice.

10 BEAUTY TIPS

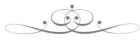

ANNA SCHARL

10 Beauty Tips

ANNA SCHARL
MAKEUP ARTIST

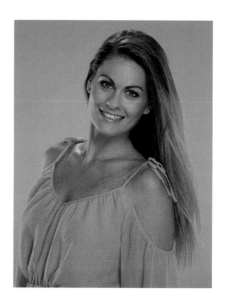

Anna Scharl has been a successful international makeup artist for 15 years. In addition to her work as a makeup artist, she is also a lecturer at various cosmetology schools. Anna Scharl's clients include major television stations and fashion labels, as well as a number of international celebrities. As a trained hair stylist, cosmetologist, and makeup artist, Anna Scharl is the perfect expert for your wedding-day beauty tips.

Good preparation is absolutely necessary for the bride to dazzle with fabulous makeup and hair styling on her big day. I have compiled a few to-dos and tips I think are important so you can fully enjoy your wedding and still look radiant all day.

NAILS

As soon as you are engaged, everyone wants to see your beautiful ring. That means your hands are constantly the center of attention. Prepare your hands and nails for all that

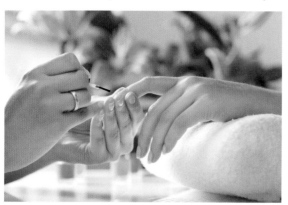

attention and keep them beautiful with weekly manicures. That is also your opportunity to experiment with colors and get to know your manicurist.

She will offer you several options to keep your nails looking perfect. In addition to traditional nail polish, there is also shellac, which lasts twice as long. Gel or acrylic nails are another even more permanent method. The difference is that acrylic nails are more resilient than gel nails and can be shaped thinner because of the harder material.

If you choose to wear open-toe shoes, I suggest painting your toenails the same color as your fingernails, and for an overall groomed look, it is important to have the calluses removed from your heels.

BODY AND SKIN

Sun-kissed skin will give you a natural and healthy appearance. You can use a bronzer, which are available as crèmes or sprays that work progressively. The sure-fire method is to go to an airbrush-tanning studio. The pros there will recommend a spray tan that matches your skin tone, ideally a few days before the wedding. That will leave some time

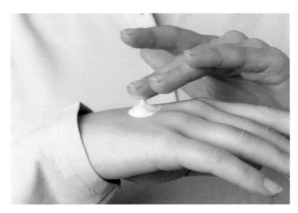

in case problem areas have to be corrected to ensure that the color looks more natural. Just one application will be enough to give you that slightly tanned look for your photos. If you are getting married in late summer, you will most likely already have a tan.

Do you have tough-to-treat trouble spots like dry elbows or knees? A body-peel (e.g., sea salt peel) in the shower will lift away dead skin cells. Afterwards, you should apply a generous amount of a rich crème or lotion to the area and allow it to absorb.

If you want to treat yourself, book a whole-body peel at a studio for beautiful skin. For instance, try a sugar peel for soft and sweet-smelling skin.

Use a shimmer body lotion on your wedding day to give your skin the perfect glow.

TEETH

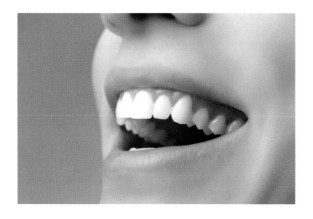

A gleaming white smile is ideal for wedding photos. Most toothpaste has whitening ingredients, but for a quicker result you can use one with a special whitening effect. White strips are another option. The more expensive but also most effective method is to get your teeth whitened professionally. Be sure to keep it natural looking, because anything that looks too artificial will be very noticeable in photos. Ideally, schedule your teeth whitening six months before the wedding and your teeth will be perfect on your big day.

MOUTH AND LIPS

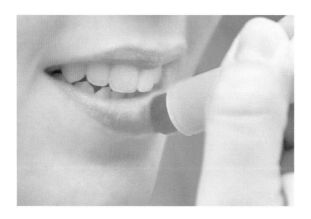

Apply lip balm or Vaseline at night a couple days before your wedding. To remove dead skin, massage your lips with a damp washcloth. For a bigger peeling effect, you can also use a toothbrush to gently brush your lips. Choose glossy lips for your wedding day. Matte lipstick is a classic look, but it doesn't last as long and becomes uneven. It is also more difficult to touch up than gloss. You can apply lip gloss over your lipstick, but there are also very glossy lipsticks.

FACE AND COSMETICS

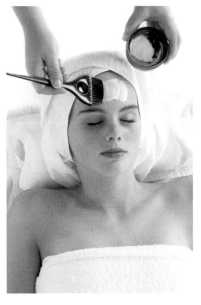

A good hydrating serum fills in wrinkles caused by dry skin and lets your skin gleam. It is best to start several weeks before the wedding. Ideally, apply the serum every morning, even under your makeup.

Do you want to treat yourself? Plan monthly facials for your bridal glow at least three months before your wedding. They promote healthy skin and make it look more clear and radiant.

Depending on skin findings, I would suggest specific beauty treatments. You might start with simple techniques like skin-refining microdermabrasion, or more elaborate methods that effectively saturate or tighten tired skin such as Mesoporation. These procedures immediately improve skin appearance and quality. The result is beautiful, even skin—a wonderful foundation for the perfect wedding makeup.

I recommend using a nice moisturizing mask the night before the wedding, preferably one you have already used to prevent possible intolerances.

EYEBROWS

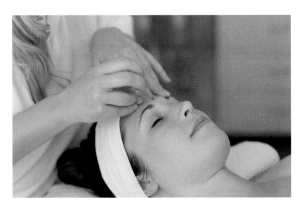

If you usually pluck your eyebrows yourself, take this opportunity and let a pro do it. An esthetician can make suggestions for the shape that best suits your face. Waxing is also an option. Eyebrow threading with cotton threads is even more precise, faster, and gentler. Here, too, I suggest starting with a professional plucking several weeks before the wedding, so on your big day the result is perfect. Please do not pluck on your wedding day to avoid unnecessary redness.

MAKEUP TRIAL

You should add a makeup trial to your hair trial at least three months before the wedding. At that time, you can discuss the details of your look and will know exactly what you will look like.

Do you want to treat yourself? Hire a photographer for a makeup shoot. You'll know exactly what your makeup will look like in your wedding photos. If the makeup looks too heavy or too light in the photos, repeat the whole thing with new makeup.

LASHES

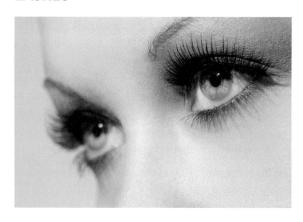

Eyelashes emphasize the eyes and, in my opinion, are an important part of a fantastic overall makeup. If yours are short, just add some false ones. There are several options.

If you want something less noticeable, you can just use half strips that attach to the outer edge of the lid and create a romantic look. My favorites are accent lashes that can be glued on individually between your own natural lashes. The glue is not permanent and your makeup pro can attach them on top of your finished makeup on your wedding day. You can simply pull them off to remove them the same day.

If you are looking for a more permanent solution, you can have extensions made at an eyelash studio. There are various methods and the pros at the studio will be happy to advise you. The application lasts until the natural lash falls out. You will need touch-ups every three to four weeks.

HAIR

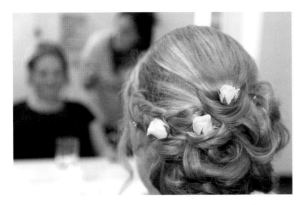

I recommend working with your stylist to come up with a hair care plan months before your wedding. You should also talk about the length of your hair for the wedding or what color you would like it to be. If you choose an updo, talk about which hair length would be most suitable for that style. And here, too, the rule is: don't wait until just before the wedding—do it months ahead of time!

How do you want to wear your hair?

Choose a hairstyle that suits your personality. Don't try to wear something particularly outrageous on your wedding day because—and you can trust me on this—when you look at your wedding photos in five years you will ask yourself who that weird-looking woman next to your husband is.

There are no rules or traditions you have to obey on your wedding day. Most important is that you don't drive yourself crazy about your hairstyle and that you feel comfortable. It's better to choose a more casual style than being too coiffed.

Important Details

I recommend hiring a makeup artist who will also fix your hair so it's all done by one person, and ideally that person will come to your home or hotel on your big day. That saves you lots of stress and time on an already hectic day. Allow enough time to change clothes and rest after your makeup appointment. Make an additional appointment 4-8 weeks before the wedding to talk about what you want and to do a trial run, so there won't be any nasty surprises on your big day.

Bring a photo of your wedding dress and the type of veil you plan to wear. Learn about current bridal hairstyles and get inspiration for your own hairstyle. Of course, your hair length and hairstyle are the determining factors:

- **Short hair.** Short hair is perfect for hair ornaments. Add gorgeous accents to your hair with flowers that match your bridal bouquet, or use a decorative comb or barrette that emphasizes your dress. Even a short haircut offers wonderful opportunities for an exceptional hairstyle.

- **Mid-length hair.** Shoulder-length hair offers lots of choices. If you want to wear your hair down, soft, loose curls or waves create a romantic look, while hair that is pinned up in a bun can be turned into an elegant updo.

- **Long hair.** Hair styles that are half pinned up and half loose, either smooth or with waves or curls are currently very popular with brides with long hair. Low buns that cover the nape or low ponytails tied with a glittery hair tie make elegant updos.

Headbands with flowers or large barrettes that hold back a section of hair are very attractive if you want to let your hair fall naturally, but wish to jazz it up a bit.

If you have a veil and plan to take it off at the reception, talk to your hair stylist and she will work it into your hairstyle so you can easily remove it yourself.

HAIR REMOVAL

A little fuzz on your upper lip is no big deal in everyday life, but you don't want to be able to see it in your wedding photos. To get the best results, start with monthly waxes as soon as possible. The chocolate wax or sugar wax methods are a little less painful. If you have long contemplated permanent hair removal via laser, now is the time to act. Prepare for your honeymoon by having those little hairs removed by laser. To be hair-free requires three treatments with one month between treatments. It takes approximately seven months for permanent results.

MAKEUP

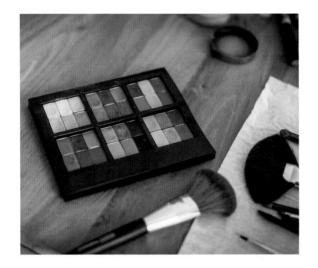

In my opinion, makeup is important because it draws attention to the bride's personality, her beauty, and her charms. When planning a wedding, most brides understandably think about the dress first when it comes to their look. But you should also find a good professional makeup artist early, because the good ones are booked months ahead of time.

A bride's makeup should primarily be appropriate for her look. You don't want something completely different on the day of the wedding. You want to look like yourself and feel comfortable. For instance, if you usually wear bright red lipstick, it should also be part of your bridal makeup. If the bride usually wears little to no makeup, it doesn't make sense to completely change her look for her wedding, unless she wishes to do so.

Most brides prefer subtle, natural-looking makeup. It is the first choice when the dress and hairstyle are very glamorous or elaborate. In this case, dramatic makeup would be too much. But a bride wearing a simple dress and a more casual hairstyle can wear more dramatic makeup to provide contrast. I recommend emphasizing either the eyes or the mouth, but there are not trends for bridal makeup.

There are, however, a few basic criteria that apply to every bride, and it is my experience that every woman likes the way they make them look.

- Eyes

Brown and pink shades in eye makeup look good on every woman and are perfectly suited to create a subtle expressive look. Adding a highlighter below the eyebrows opens up the eyes. The eyebrows should definitely be emphasized, which makes the eyes even more expressive and more of an eye-catcher in the wedding photos. Waterproof mascara is a must in case those tears of joy begin to fall. I recommend to my clients to only dab at their tears rather than wiping them off.

- **Complexion**

A bride's face is often covered with too much foundation out of fear that the skin won't look perfect enough in the wedding photos or won't be covered well enough all day. If you have some moles or blemishes, cover them beforehand (e.g., with a concealer) and keep the foundation light. Too much foundation settles in wrinkles, which makes you look unnecessarily older. There are some great products by various makeup brands that look light and radiant on the skin.

I like to use highlighters on top of blush and on the bridge of the nose to create luster and make the face look fresh and radiant.

- **Lips**

Use a lip balm in advance to moisturize your lips and make them smooth and soft. I like using lip liner. It makes lipstick last longer and keeps it from bleeding into the small wrinkles around the mouth. Subtle shades of pink or coral look good on any woman and are easier to touch up than bold shades of red. Often a little lip gloss is enough to bring some color and shine to your lips.

- **Eyebrows**

Eyebrows can make the difference between a positive and negative facial appearance. They shape the face. It is best to lightly trace them with an eyebrow pencil. Eyebrow powder has a more natural effect. There are also amazing eyebrow mascaras that can be used to fix the eyebrows in place.

Brides should avoid too much luster and glitter in the face. It makes the complexion look too greasy in photos taken with a strong flash. The risk of makeup mishaps can be largely avoided if the makeup artist responds to the bride's personality and a rehearsal appointment is scheduled in advance.

The maid-of-honor helps with touching up the makeup in-between, at most with powder, lipstick, or gloss. So-called *blotter paper* that soaks up excess skin oil and a few cotton swabs (in case the makeup does get out of place) should be in your purse. If you have an updo, you should also have a few bobby pins on hand in case this or that strand of hair gets loose. I also recommend a mini hairspray.

The makeup appointment is the beginning of an eventful day for every bride. Often, photos are taken during the makeup session. Here are a few tips for creating an awesome set that I have picked up during my work with many different brides over the course of my career:

- To avoid too much excitement and fuss, make sure that only the people closest to you attend your makeup and hair-styling session.

- During her styling appointment, the bride can wear a nice satin robe with the word *Bride* on the back in rhinestones. To make it even cuter, add some slippers with the word *Bride* or something similar on the soles. If that is too much, just wear a simple soft white top or dress. I think it's fun when the bride is dressed in white during her makeup session.

- One bride had a custom perfume bottle created that had hers and her husband's name on the label.

- The bridal gown can already be hung in the room on a nice wooden—preferably white—hanger, possibly with the word *Bride* on it.

- Beautiful flowers and candles in the room make for a festive atmosphere. Playing the bride's favorite music will help lighten up the generally nervous, tense vibe in the room.

- I personally love balloons in pastel colors and think it's great when there are some in the room during the makeup appointment. Wooden letters spelling out "Mr. & Mrs." are also a fun idea.

- A chilled bottle of Prosecco in a nice cooler is a must-have, but the makeup artist should not imbibe too much.

In summary, preparation is everything! Good planning prevents unnecessary hassles and lets the big day turn into a relaxed event.

For the day after the wedding, I would recommend a cooling eye mask, lots of moisturizing face cream, aspirin, and lots of water.

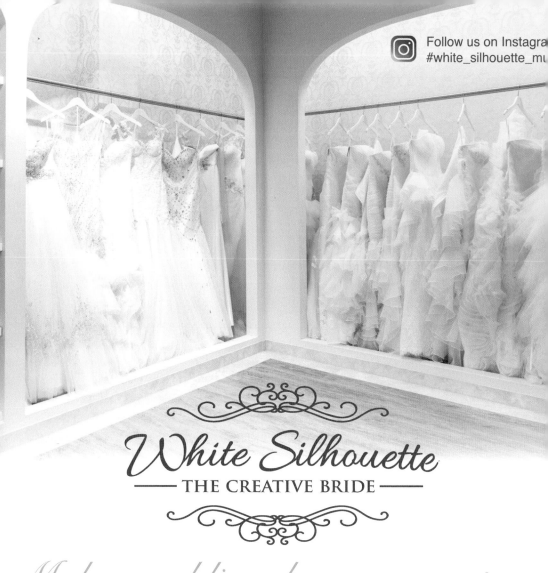